Successful Randomized Trials

Successful Randomized Trials
A Handbook for the 21st Century

EDITED BY

Michael J. Domanski, MD
Chief, Atherothrombosis and Coronary Artery Disease Branch
National Heart, Lung, and Blood Institute
Bethesda, Maryland
USA

Sonja McKinlay, PhD
President
New England Research Institutes, Inc.
Watertown, Massachusetts
USA

Wolters Kluwer | Lippincott Williams & Wilkins
Health
Philadelphia · Baltimore · New York · London
Buenos Aires · Hong Kong · Sydney · Tokyo

Acquisitions Editor: Frances R. DeStefano
Managing Editor: Leanne McMillan
Project Manager: Jennifer Harper
Senior Manufacturing Manager: Benjamin Rivera
Marketing Manager: Kimberly S. Schonberger
Design Coordinator: Terry Mallon
Production Services: International Typesetting and Composition

© 2009 by LIPPINCOTT WILLIAMS & WILKINS, a Wolters Kluwer business

530 Walnut Street
Philadelphia, PA 19106 USA
LWW.com

All rights reserved. This book is protected by copyright. No part of this book may be reproduced in any form by any means, including photocopying, or utilized by any information storage and retrieval system without written permission from the copyright owner, except for brief quotations embodied in critical articles and reviews. Materials appearing in this book prepared by individuals as part of their official duties as U.S. government employees are not covered by the above-mentioned copyright.

Printed in China
Library of Congress Cataloging-in-Publication Data

Successful randomized trials : a handbook for the 21st century / [edited by] Michael J. Domanski, Sonja McKinlay.
  p. ; cm.
  Includes bibliographical references and index.
  ISBN-13: 978-0-7817-7945-6
  ISBN-10: 0-7817-7945-6
  1. Clinical trials. I. Domanski, Michael J. II. McKinlay, Sonja.
  [DNLM: 1. Randomized Controlled Trials as Topic. QV 771 S942 2009]
  R853.C55S83 2009
  610.72'4—dc22

2008033571

Care has been taken to confirm the accuracy of the information presented and to describe generally accepted practices. However, the authors, editors, and publisher are not responsible for errors or omissions or for any consequences from application of the information in this book and make no warranty, expressed or implied, with respect to the currency, completeness, or accuracy of the contents of the publication. Application of the information in a particular situation remains the professional responsibility of the practitioner.

The authors, editors, and publisher have exerted every effort to ensure that drug selection and dosage set forth in this text are in accordance with current recommendations and practice at the time of publication. However, in view of ongoing research, changes in government regulations, and the constant flow of information relating to drug therapy and drug reactions, the reader is urged to check the package insert for each drug for any change in indications and dosage and for added warnings and precautions. This is particularly important when the recommended agent is a new or infrequently employed drug.

Some drugs and medical devices presented in the publication have Food and Drug Administration (FDA) clearance for limited use in restricted research settings. It is the responsibility of the health care provider to ascertain the FDA status of each drug or device planned for use in their clinical practice.

To purchase additional copies of this book, call our customer service department at (800) 638-3030 or fax orders to (301) 223-2320. International customers should call (301) 223-2300.

Visit Lippincott Williams & Wilkins on the Internet: at LWW.com. Lippincott Williams & Wilkins customer service representatives are available from 8:30 am to 6 pm, EST.

10 9 8 7 6 5 4 3 2 1

To my Mother and Father, Beatrice and Thaddeus Domanski, whose love and guidance made all things possible for me; and to my sons, David and Daniel, who make my world complete.

MJD

To the memory of Bill (WG) Cochran, for whom clarity was a driving force; and to life partner and closest colleague, John McKinlay, whose extensive contributions to science and policy have always exemplified the essential role of well-designed experiments.

SMK

CONTENTS

Contributors ix
Preface xi
Foreword xiii
Abbreviations xv

SECTION I
Clinical Trial Principles

1. Randomized Clinical Trials 3
   MICHAEL J. DOMANSKI AND SONJA MCKINLAY

2. Designing Clinical Trials 5
   SUSAN F. ASSMANN

3. Randomization: What It Is and How to Do It 27
   CATHERINE E. HEWITT AND DAVID J. TORGERSON

4. Setting Sample Size for Randomized Clinical Trials 45
   XIN TIAN, SONJA M. MCKINLAY, AND NANCY L. GELLER

5. Analytic Approach and Methods 71
   LYNN A. SLEEPER

6. Ethical Considerations 101
   LAWRENCE M. FRIEDMAN AND ELEANOR B. SCHRON

SECTION II
Large Multicenter Trials: Structure and Conduct

7. Study Organization and Governance 119
   FLEUR HUDSON, JULIE BAKOBAKI, AND ABDEL BABIKER

8. Quality Control and Quality Assurance 141
   FLORA S. SIAMI

9. Quality Assurance: Prevention of Missing Data 151
   JAMES NEATON

vii

SECTION III
The Future

10. Surrogate Endpoints 167
ROBERT FIORENTINO

11. Registries 173
HESHA DUGGIRALA

12. Gazing into the Crystal Ball: The Future of
Randomized Clinical Trials 179
MICHAEL J. DOMANSKI, SONJA M. MCKINLAY, AND MARC PFEFFER

Index   191

Contributors

Susan F. Assmann, PhD
New England Research Institutes
Watertown, Massachusetts
USA

Abdel Babiker
Head
HIV and Infections Group
MRC Clinical Trials Unit
London, United Kingdom

Julie Bakobaki
Clinical Project Manager
MRC Clinical Trials Unit
London, United Kingdom

Michael J. Domanski, MD
Chief, Atherothrombosis and
Coronary Artery Disease Branch
National Heart, Lung, and Blood
Institute
Bethesda, Maryland
USA

Hesha J. Duggirala, PhD
Epidemiologist
Office of Surveillance and Biometrics
Center for Devices and
Radiological Health
Food and Drug Administration
Chevy Chase, Maryland
USA

Robert P. Fiorentino, MD, MPH
U.S. Food and Drug
Administration
Bethesda, Maryland
USA

Lawrence M. Friedman, MD
Independent Consultant
Rockville, Maryland
USA

Nancy L. Geller
Director, Office of Biostatistics
Research
National Heart, Lung, and Blood
Institute
National Institutes of Health
Bethesda, Maryland
USA

Catherine E. Hewitt, MD
Research Fellow
Department of Health Sciences
University of York
Heslington, United Kingdom

Fleur Hudson
Clinical Operations Manager
MRC (Medical Research
Council) Clinical Trials Unit
London, United Kingdom

Sonja M. McKinlay, PhD
President
New England Research Institutes, Inc.
Watertown, Massachusetts
USA

James Neaton
Professor
Division of Biostatistics
School of Public Health
University of Minnesota
Minneapolis, Minnesota
USA

Marc A. Pfeffer, MD, PhD
Dzau Professor of Medicine
Harvard Medical School
Cardiovascular Division
Brigham and Women's Hospital
Cardiovascular Division
Brigham and Women's Hospital
Boston, Massachusetts
USA

Eleanor B. Schron, PhD, RN
Program Director
Atherothrombosis and Coronary
Artery Disease Branch
Division of Cardiovascular Diseases
National Heart, Lung, and Blood
Institute
National Institutes of Health
Bethesda, Maryland
USA

Flora Sandra Siami, MPH, RAC
Director
Regulatory Affairs
Principal Research Scientist
New England Research Institutes
Watertown, Massachusetts
USA

Lynn A. Sleeper, ScD
Chief Scientist
New England Research Institutes, Inc.
Watertown, Massachusetts
USA

Xin Tian, PhD
Mathematical Statistician
Office of Biostatistics Research
National Heart, Lung, and Blood
Institute
National Institutes of Health
Bethesda, Maryland
USA

David J. Torgerson
Director, York Trials Unit
Department of Health Sciences
University of York
York, United Kingdom

PREFACE

Our vision for this volume is that it be useful both as a text for introductory courses on randomized controlled trials in Medical Schools, Schools of Nursing, and Schools of Public Health and as a handy resource for the successful design and conduct of randomized trials.

The chapters in this text convey the accumulated wisdom of leading international clinical trialists representing a broad range of experience. Our goal is to present this knowledge—both theoretical and practical—in a user-friendly, helpful handbook that will become a well thumbed friend on the shelf—even in this electronic era! Examples, illustrations, and handy checklists abound. Anything resembling formulas is intentionally absent. Practical information, seldom found in published material, is evident throughout the handbook.

Organized in three sections, the Handbook first leads the reader through all the key considerations in designing a randomized controlled trial (six Chapters in Section I). Three Chapters in Section II present invaluable practical information that is seldom available for implementing a successful trial. In the final Section, three short Chapters focus on emerging issues and provide a provocative glimpse of future randomized trials in the electronic 21st Century.

We particularly wish to acknowledge the extraordinary effort of our contributors, in the midst of their very busy lives managing large, international multi-site trials, who took the time to articulate their considerable experience in a novel and accessible way—an exercise requiring considerably more effort and thought than a technical chapter in a standard textbook! Their suggestions for further (more technical) reading also required thoughtful choices. They made our job as co-editors remarkably easy.

Michael J. Domanski
Sonja McKinlay

FOREWORD

Randomized clinical trials are the cornerstone for rational decision-making in medicine. Yet the principles and methods governing the design, organization, and conduct of clinical trials remain largely enigmatic for a broad spectrum of persons, ranging from biomedical professionals to current and potential research subjects (i.e., the public). Virtually every day, the press hails another "landmark" clinical trial, or, alternatively, decries another fiasco resulting from an impropriety in the conduct of biomedical research. Significant effort and time will be needed if clinical trials are to be understood in their proper perspective—as fundamental tools for building, piece by small piece, a framework of knowledge that can ultimately be used to guide clinical decision-making.

In recent years, concepts such as evidence-based medicine, quality measurement, and learning health systems have been established as overarching conceptual frameworks capable of providing direction to the delivery of health care. However, trying to develop and implement these constructs without the basic knowledge provided by randomized clinical trials would be tantamount to erecting a skyscraper without a firm foundation. Despite this, relatively little attention has been devoted to the question of how clinical trials can be made more successful in terms of quality and efficiency.

The past decade has witnessed the increasing industrialization of clinical trials. In the 1970s, clinical studies were largely the preserve of academic medical centers and were typically funded by the National Institutes of Health. As learning progressed from these early experiences, clinical outcomes trials grew in size due to the realization that treatment effects are usually modest; at the same time, biological proof-of-concept trials became more expensive and resource-intensive as scientific technology underwent a series of revolutionary changes. Additionally, as consensus emerged regarding the desirability of requiring proof of efficacy to support the proper labeling of medical drugs and devices, the U.S. Food and Drug Administration began to demand more trials with higher levels of quality from the medical products industry.

These demands resulted in a number of positive outcomes: many trials are now global in extent, practice and research communities are involved in almost every sector of health care, and there is a general expectation that practice will be based on the best available evidence. Far less desirable, however, are dramatic increases in the costs and bureaucratic entanglements attendant upon clinical research. These increases have been particularly notable in the United States, where current surveys point to a decline in investigators participating in trials at the very time that their importance is gaining widespread recognition.

It is for these reasons that I was especially pleased when Drs. Domanski and McKinlay asked me to write the foreword for *Successful Clinical Trials*—a book both timely and important. These two researchers are giants in the theory and practice of clinical trials: Dr. Domanski is both a practicing clinician and a leader at the National Heart, Lung and Blood Institute, while Dr. McKinlay runs a highly successful clinical trials coordinating center. Together with their friends and colleagues, they have succeeded in writing a book whose distilled experience and understanding reflects the simplicity and profundity of the title. The chapter authors are distinguished clinician-scientists who have conducted successful trials—people who can "walk the walk" as well as "talk the talk."

Successful Clinical Trials addresses the broad fundamentals of clinical trials in three domains: principles, operations, and innovation. The first section, Clinical Trials Principles, introduces the reader to the basics of trial design, concepts of randomization, and statistical analysis, as well as addressing pragmatic ethical issues and organizational and decision-making constructs. The second section, which specifically addresses large multicenter trials, is particularly useful in enabling the reader to discern the differences between truly important, sensible aspects of trial design and conduct, as distinct from the accretions of largely unnecessary bureaucratic impedimenta, whose contributions to higher quality are dubious at best. Finally, the book explores issues critical to the future of clinical research: What should we make of the current focus on surrogate endpoints and biomarkers? How can we use registries to complement and enhance clinical trials? What major changes can we foresee as technological enhancements, restructuring of the healthcare system, and globalization of biomedical research continue to evolve?

This book is an essential primer for those seeking an introduction to the truly essential concepts of clinical trials, while its references point to a comprehensive array of detailed reading for those who want to dig deeper. Readers who absorb the messages contained in this book and employ these key concepts in clinical research and practice will be doing the world a great service, as together we continue to add to the knowledge that makes possible the prevention and treatment of disease through the conduct of successful clinical trials.

Robert M. Califf, MD, MACC
Vice Chancellor for Clinical Research
Duke University Medical Center
Director, Duke Translational Medicine Institute

Abbreviations

ACCORD	Action to Control Cardiovascular Risk in Diabetics
A-HeFT	African-American Heart Failure
CAPA	Corrective and Preventive Action
CATCH	Child and Adolescent Trial for Cardiovascular Health
CEC	Clinical Events Committee
CIOMS	Council for International Organizations of Medical Sciences
CONSENSE II	Cooperative New Scandinavian Enalapril Survival Study II
CONVINCE	Controlled Onset Investigation of Cardiovascular End Points
CQI	Continuous Quality Improvement
CRF	Case report form
CTAs	Clinical Trial Authorizations
DASH	Dietary Approaches to Stop Hypertension
DMC	Data Monitoring Committee
DSMB	Data Safety and Monitoring Board
EU	European Union
FDA	Food and Drug Administration
FWA	Federal Wide Assurance
GCP	Good Clinical Practice
ICH	International Conference on Harmonization
IDE	Investigational Device Exemption
IMP	Investigational Medicinal Product
IND	Investigational New Drug
INSIGHT	International Network for Strategic Initiatives in Global HIV Trials
ITT	Intention to Treat
JAMA	Journal of the American Medical Association
MAGIC	Magnesium in Coronaries Study
NIH	National Institutes of Health
OCC	Overall Coordinating Center

PEACE	Prevention of Events with Angiotensin-Converting Enzyme Inhibition
PICO	Pimobendam in Congestive Heart Failure
PLADO	Platelet Dose Study
PT	Protocol Team
QA, QC	Quality assurance, control
QOL	Quality-of-Life
RCTs	Randomized Controlled Trials
SAS	Statistical Analysis System
SDV	Source document verification
SOPs	Standard operating procedures
TMG	Trial Management Group
TSC	Trial Steering Committee
VAlHeft	Valsartan Heart Failure Trial

Successful Randomized Trials
A Handbook for the 21st Century

SECTION I

Clinical Trial Principles

Randomized Clinical Trials

MICHAEL J. DOMANSKI • SONJA M. MCKINLAY

Implicit in the modern practice of medicine is the use of therapies scientifically proven to be effective. Where the natural history of a disease can be predicted with certainty, simply observing the effect of a treatment being studied on a group of patients would provide the needed assessment. Most often, however, the disease course is not sufficiently predictable for such an observational study to be useful. Additionally, the size of the expected effect of many treatments is small enough that separating treatment effect from the play of chance is only feasible in randomized controlled trials (RCTs).

Randomized controlled trials are not new; a comparison of the effect of different diets on young palace servants is recorded in the Bible in the Book of Daniel. One might, however, question whether the palace servants were indeed comparable at the start of the study at baseline, because differences in their constitution might have been the reason for the apparent difference in outcome. This limitation can be obviated by randomly assigning subjects to different study groups, generating what is referred to as an RCT.

Randomized controlled trials are experiments in which individuals are randomly assigned to different treatments and then the results are compared with respect to a predefined endpoint. Randomization is central to producing a scientifically valid study. Randomizing subjects is the best way to maximize the chance that individuals assigned to different treatment groups are comparable at the start of the study. By "comparable," we mean that biases, recognized and unrecognized, that could influence trial outcome independent of the treatment, are absent.

The RCT has become the foundation of evidence-based medical practice. The approach to conducting these studies has matured in ways that provide a substantial assurance of methodologic validity and ethical conduct.

This book is intended, first and foremost, to provide the background and practical knowledge needed for medical professionals to actually engage in and conduct large clinical trials. Throughout, we have studiously sacrificed rigor for clarity, making the text accessible to individuals with limited mathematical training. The text is divided into three sections.

Section I is devoted to the scientific and methodologic basis of RCTs. Fundamental concepts are presented, including the following:

1. Trial design
   - *Selection of an appropriate cohort of subjects.* Essential in this regard is selecting patients for entry into the trial who are indeed representative of the general patient population for whom the treatment is intended.
   - *Choice of an appropriate endpoint.* The endpoint should be clinically important and nonbiased ascertainment of its occurrence should be feasible. Combined endpoints must be carefully crafted to include components of comparable clinical importance.
   - *Defining a clinically relevant effect.* A treatment studied in an RCT should promise the possibility of sufficient therapeutic effect to be clinically relevant. That is, there should be the expectation that clinical practice would be meaningfully guided by the result.
2. Randomization
   - Subjectivity in choice of treatment must be eliminated.
3. Setting sample size
   - An RCT should be of sufficient size and have a sufficient number of events to yield not only a qualitative result but also a robust quantitative estimate of effect size and complication rate.
4. Statistical analysis plan
   - *Prospective protocol development.* A statistical analysis plan, including primary, secondary, and subgroup analyses, must be prespecified to avoid subjective choice of findings. Clear guidelines for early stopping (for safety, effectiveness, or futility) are also required.
5. Assuring adequate protection of trial subjects. To ensure safety and ethnical conduct, monitoring by an independent body, throughout the trial, is required.

Section II, composed of three chapters, provides practical information that is seldom available, especially in print. Although there is no substitute for experience, these "how to" chapters provide a handy blueprint for how to design and implement a successful trial while avoiding major pitfalls.

Section III, with three chapters, covers emerging topics related to clinical trials methodology and the current and future role of clinical trials.

CHAPTER 2

Designing Clinical Trials

SUSAN F. ASSMANN

This chapter discusses various clinical trial designs, emphasizing Phase III randomized controlled trials. Selecting the appropriate trial design depends, first of all, on clearly specifying the research question to be answered. This is the subject of the first section.

The second section discusses issues related to blinding of trials—that is, concealing which treatment is being assigned.

The most common study designs, and when to consider each type of design, are described in the third section.

Issues regarding what proportion of subjects (or other experimental units) to assign to each treatment group are discussed in the fourth section.

SPECIFYING THE RESEARCH QUESTION

The first step in designing a clinical trial is to clearly specify the primary research question. A number of issues should be considered (see box). Careful consideration of these issues is necessary in selecting the optimal design and creating a study protocol.

Of course, the data collected in the study may be used to answer additional prespecified research questions, or to carry out additional exploratory analyses that may guide the design of future studies. However, there is a single question (occasionally two) for which trial design must assure adequate statistical power. Trying to design a study to answer too many questions at once can result in a larger, more complex study that may prove difficult to carry out and interpret.

> **SPECIFYING THE RESEARCH QUESTION**
>
> The following issues must all be addressed to clearly specify the research question:
>
> - What phase is the study?
> - What treatment strategies will be studied?
> - How will the primary outcome be defined and measured?
> - What subject population will be studied?
> - What is the unit of analysis?
> - Is the goal to show that A is better than B? Noninferior to B? Equivalent to B?

Study Phases

Clinical trials are often categorized as Phase I, Phase II, Phase III, or Phase IV.

- A Phase I trial investigates the pharmacokinetics of a drug—how it is distributed through the body, its metabolism, and its toxicities. Often a Phase I trial involves dose-finding, that is, establishing what dose can be tolerated without excessive toxicity. Phase I studies are usually not randomized.
- A Phase II trial looks for preliminary evidence that the treatment has some clinical efficacy. A Phase II trial may or may not be randomized. Data are also collected about the safety of the treatment.
- A Phase III trial compares two or more treatment strategies (one of which may be placebo treatment or no treatment). Phase III trials are generally randomized. This book concentrates on Phase III randomized clinical trials.
- A Phase IV trial is a surveillance study in a large group of subjects, to estimate the frequency of side effects, interactions with other medications, and so forth, when the treatment is used in actual clinical practice. Usually Phase III trials do not enroll enough subjects to discover uncommon side effects or interactions. Phase IV studies are usually not randomized.

Some studies combine more than one phase.

Choice of Treatment Strategies

Most randomized clinical trials include two treatment strategies, although studies can include three or more. Examples of treatment strategies include medications, devices, surgical interventions, behavioral interventions, and combinations of interventions. Treatment strategies can also include placebo treatment, or even no treatment at all.

Often there is one "investigational" treatment, and the goal of the study is to compare this new treatment strategy with a "control" treatment strategy. The control treatment strategy can be a treatment in current use, placebo, or no treatment. The rest of this section assumes this general study design, but similar considerations apply to other types of studies.

Specification of the Investigational Treatment

Usually it is clear from the outset what investigational treatment will be studied, such as a newly developed medication, an existing medication that may be useful for a new indication, a new medical device, a new procedure, or a lifestyle intervention. Sometimes there are other issues that may be relevant to consider. How will the medication be dosed (including methods for dose modification, if relevant)? What formulation will be used? For example, some medications may be given either orally or intravenously. Will a particular brand be used, or are all brands considered equivalent? For example, different brands of warfarin may have different effects at the same dose, but different brands of aspirin may be considered equivalent to each other.

Active Control

For some studies, it may not be ethical to have one treatment strategy consist of a placebo treatment or no treatment. This is especially the case for a study involving a serious condition for which at least one active treatment is available and known to have some benefit. Even if there is no treatment that has been proven efficacious, there may be a treatment that is commonly used. Subjects or referring physicians may be uncomfortable agreeing to a study in which the control group goes without this active treatment.

If the control strategy is to involve active treatment, a decision must be made about how strictly the protocol should specify this treatment. The possibilities range from an "anything goes" approach (so long as it does not involve the experimental treatment), to specifying exactly what treatment will be given, exactly how initial dosing and dose changes will be determined, or exactly how procedures will be carried out. The more strictly defined the control treatment is, the clearer and more interpretable the comparison will be between the experimental treatment and the control treatment. There will be less variability within the control group, so sample size may be decreased. On the other hand, there may be a risk of specifying the control treatment so narrowly that physicians may be unwilling to participate in the study or refer subjects to it. In addition, a control treatment may be so narrowly specified that it bears little relationship to actual clinical practice, resulting in a study with a clear comparison that is not clinically relevant (Fig. 2.1).

Another decision to be made, for studies with an active control, is whether the experimental treatment strategy should consist only of the experimental medication/device/procedure or whether it should include the experimental treatment in addition to the control treatment. Often this choice will be clear. A subject can receive an experimental artificial heart valve or a standard artificial heart valve, but not both. On the other hand, it would not be reasonable to treat neutropenic subjects with a serious infection only by transfusing granulocytes while withholding all other antimicrobial therapies.

Narrow Definition
- Clearer, more interpretable comparisons
- Less variability within group, possibly lower sample size

Broad Definition
- More similar to actual clinical practice
- More palatable to referring physicians

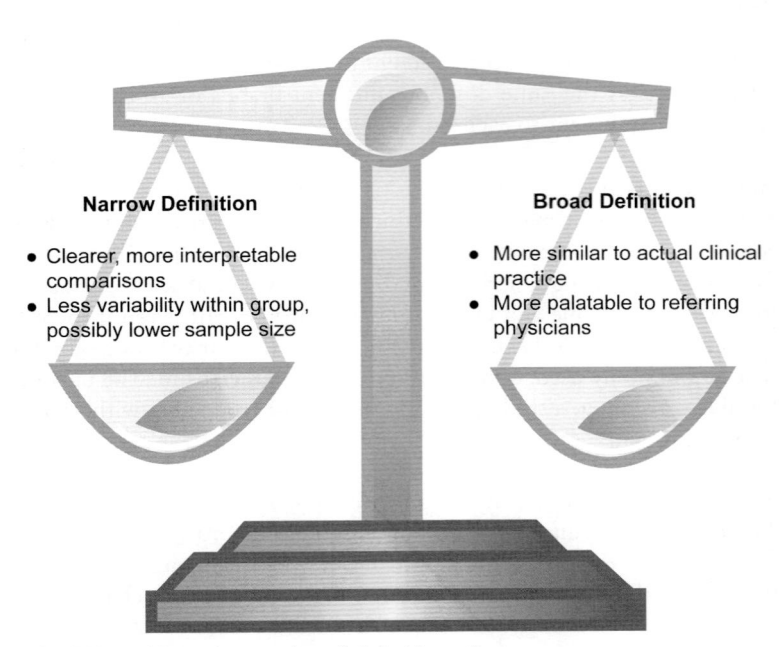

FIGURE 2.1 Narrow versus broad definition of treatment.

Placebo Control Versus No-Treatment Control

For studies that do not involve an active control, a decision must be made about whether to use a placebo treatment or no treatment at all. Considerations include the following:

- Need for blinding of treatment assignment.
- Risks of placebo treatment.
- Feasibility of placebo treatment.

Many trials involve blinding, that is, concealing which treatment is being given. This can reduce bias in the assessment of subjective outcomes, and bias in which subjects are assigned to which treatment group. (Blinding is discussed further in the next section of this chapter.) If it is necessary to blind which treatment is being given, then a no-treatment strategy is not an option since it would be clear whether a subject is being given no treatment or some treatment.

Sometimes a placebo treatment may involve some risk to the subjects. For oral medications, this is not usually much of an issue. However, if the investigational treatment is a surgical intervention, sham surgery may involve anesthetic use, or an actual incision, either of which carries some risk. Generally, sham operations are regarded as unethical. If the experimental treatment is an IV medication, and the subjects would not normally have an IV line placed, then a line placement and infusion of a placebo such as saline may carry some risk.

The feasibility of placebo treatment should also be considered. If the active study treatment involves subject-specific dosing or dose titration, placebo treatment may be challenging. For example, the starting dose of prednisone can be anywhere from 5 to 60 mg/day, and the dose must be tapered rather than stopped abruptly. Prednisone tablets are available in many different doses. With open-label treatment it may be easy to provide the correct dose for each subject on each day, by using different dose tablets for different subjects or for the same subject on different days. For a placebo-controlled trial, placebo controls would need to be created for each type of tablet being used in the active treatment group.

Definition of the Primary Study Outcome

The definition of the primary study outcome is of paramount importance in designing a trial. This definition should include:

- What outcome will be considered primary.
- How will the outcome be defined.

- What data will be collected to determine the outcome.
- Over what time period will the outcome be measured.

Types of Outcome Variables

The most common types of outcome variables, from the perspective of study design and analysis, are:

- Binary (yes/no) (e.g., vital status 1 year after randomization, clearance of infection).
- Ordered categorical (e.g., level of pain—none, mild, moderate, severe).
- Continuous (e.g., LDL cholesterol, time to walk 0.1 miles).
- Time to event (e.g., time to death, time to myocardial infarction).
- Count (e.g., number of hospitalizations in 1 year after randomization).
- Rate (e.g., number of hospitalizations per month of follow-up time).
- Repeated measure (e.g., how fast weight increases from birth to 1 year, with weight measured monthly).

Choosing the Primary Study Outcome

For some studies, the outcome will be obvious. For example, if the study is to investigate a new medication to treat fever, then body temperature is likely to be the primary study outcome. For other studies, there may be several reasonable choices for what outcome to consider as the primary study outcome.

Points to consider when choosing among possible study outcomes include:

- Clinical relevance.
- Sensitivity of the outcome to the treatments being studied.
- Ability to measure the outcome in a valid and reliable way.
- Whether the outcome measure is objective or can be independently assessed, so that subjectivity can be reduced or eliminated.
- Implications for sample size.

Surrogate Outcomes

Sometimes it is not feasible to use the most clinically relevant outcome as the primary study outcome. For example, it may take a long time to occur, it may occur rarely, or it may require an invasive, risky, or expensive procedure to measure. It may be possible to use a surrogate outcome instead, such as HIV viral load for a medication to treat AIDS, or glomerular filtration rate for a treatment to prevent renal failure.

EXAMPLE 1

MAGIC: The Magnesium in Coronaries (MAGIC) study was an international large simple trial to investigate the use of magnesium sulfate (in addition to standard care) for subjects with acute myocardial infarction.[1,2] Some possible options for the primary study outcome included:

- All-cause mortality.
- Cardiovascular mortality.

Both outcomes are clinically important. Magnesium sulfate was not expected to have a high rate of life-threatening side effects, so including noncardiovascular deaths might "muddy the water" by including outcomes upon which the treatment might have no effect. On the other hand, defining and enforcing standardized definitions of cardiovascular mortality in a large international study might be challenging, and adjudication of all deaths would have added substantially to the cost of the trial. The decision was made to use all-cause mortality as the primary study outcome, because this outcome is free of subjectivity and is standard internationally.

EXAMPLE 2

PLADO: The Platelet Dose (PLADO) study, recently carried out by the Transfusion Medicine and Hemostasis Clinical Trials Network, compared different platelet dosing strategies for thrombocytopenic patients (patients with low platelet counts). Is the typical dose optimal? Or is it better to give smaller doses of platelets more often? Or is it better to give larger doses less often? Some possible options for the primary study outcome might include:

- Bleeding.
- Cost of platelet transfusions (both the cost of the platelet products, and the labor cost per transfusion).
- Cost-effectiveness.

Clearly bleeding is of clinical relevance, while cost and cost-effectiveness have major implications for health care practice. The decision was made to use bleeding as the primary study outcome, but to include key components of cost, based on the total number of platelets transfused per subject (product) and the number of platelet transfusion orders per subject (labor), as prespecified key secondary outcomes.

A good surrogate outcome should be correlated with the clinical outcome of interest both qualitatively and quantitatively. The treatment's proposed mechanism of action for the clinical outcome should be measurable by its effect on the surrogate outcome.

Even with the best knowledge available at the time of study design, using a surrogate outcome can produce incorrect results. For example, ventricular arrhythmia is correlated with sudden death. However, the Cardiac Arrythmia Suppression Trial (CAST) trial showed that certain medications expected to reduce ventricular arrhythmia did reduce it, but nevertheless were associated with *increased* mortality.[3]

Composite Outcomes

If the most clinically relevant outcome takes too long to occur, or occurs rarely, a composite outcome may provide a good solution. For example, the most relevant outcome may be death from heart failure, but a study may use a composite of death from heart failure and hospitalization due to heart failure instead. A subject who had either one of these events occur would be considered to have been a failure for the primary outcome.

Using a composite outcome often reduces the necessary sample size or the follow-up time necessary for a study. On the other hand, secondary analyses should be used to determine whether the direction of the study effect seems similar among all components of the composite outcome. For example, suppose one treatment group has a much higher proportion of subjects experiencing the primary outcome, but the difference is entirely due to a difference in heart failure hospitalizations, with no indication of any treatment effect on heart failure death. In such a situation, interpretation of the primary outcome may be problematic.

Defining the Primary Study Outcome

After the primary outcome of the study has been decided upon, there may still be questions about exactly how it should be defined. All-cause mortality needs no further definition, but for other endpoints, careful definition is necessary.

Sometimes there are different scales for measuring an outcome. For example, there are a number of different quality-of-life (QOL) scales that could be used for a study with QOL as the primary or secondary outcome.

Sometimes there are different ways that a given outcome could be analyzed. For example, suppose the clinical outcome of interest is all-cause mortality. Should the primary study outcome be a binary variable, such as dead or alive at 1 year after randomization? Or should it be a time-to-event outcome with a fixed follow-up time per subject, such as time to death, truncated for subjects still alive at 1 year after randomization? Or should it be a time-to-event outcome with some minimum follow-up for the last subject enrolled, and all subjects followed until the end of the study (e.g., time to death), censored for subjects still alive 1 year after the last subject was randomized? The choice will depend on multiple factors. These may include the time period over which the treatment is expected to have an effect, the expected rate of study enrollment, the resources that can be devoted to follow-up of subjects, and how precisely the time of the event can be measured. Usually a time-to-event design will be more statistically efficient than a binary outcome design. (See Chapter 4 for a discussion of this point.)

As another example, suppose the clinical outcome in a study of a new anti-hypertension medication is systolic blood pressure. Should the outcome be a continuous variable (e.g., the follow-up systolic blood pressure value, or the change in systolic blood pressure from the pre-randomization value)? Should it be a binary variable (e.g., whether or not the follow-up systolic blood pressure is lower than 120 mm Hg)? Usually a study with a continuous outcome will be statistically more efficient than a study that uses a binary version of the continuous outcome. (See Chapter 4 for a discussion of this point.) On the other hand, sometimes what is clinically most relevant is whether a parameter is

---

EXAMPLE 2 **(Continued)**

PLADO: There is no single validated outcome definition to measure bleeding. One commonly used scale to measure bleeding is the WHO Bleeding Scale, which gives definitions of bleeding severity for each of several body systems (oropharyngeal, gastrointestinal, etc.) and overall.[4] However, there are many aspects of bleeding, including frequency, severity, which (and how many) body systems are bleeding, and so on.[5] If a patient has grade 2 bleeding on June 1 and 2, is it feasible to determine whether these are two separate bleeding episodes or one continuous bleeding episode? Is it worse to have grade 3 bleeding in one body system for 1 day, or to have grade 2 bleeding in multiple body systems for 7 days? The decision was made to use a binary outcome, whether or not each subject had any grade 2 or higher bleeding while on study, as the primary study outcome. The highest grade of bleeding while on study was prespecified as a key secondary outcome. Other analyses of bleeding will be more exploratory in nature.

within the normal range, rather than its precise value. In addition, reliable measurement of blood pressure requires the use of calibrated automated devices and technician training.

Time Period for Measuring the Primary Study Outcome

Some studies are expected to show an effect in the short term, if they show an effect at all. This is often the case when the treatment being studied is a single intervention event for an acute condition. Other studies may only show an effect over longer periods of time. For example, the study may involve long-term treatment for a chronic condition. In some studies, one treatment group may tend to experience clinical events early in the study while the other treatment group may tend to experience clinical events over a longer period. This could occur if one treatment involves surgical intervention, which for some subjects may result in immediate clinical complications or death, while the other treatment involves a drug intervention.

Data Collection to Determine the Primary Study Outcome

Often there will be several choices of what data, and how much data, will be collected to determine the primary study outcome. Some options may

---

EXAMPLE 1 (Continued)

MAGIC: The study intervention (magnesium sulfate or placebo infusion) took place over the first 24 hours that the patient was in the study, shortly after the myocardial infarction occurred. The postulated mechanisms of effect would have occurred in the short term. The decision was made to have the primary outcome be 30-day mortality.

EXAMPLE 2 (Continued)

PLADO: The study interventions were only feasible to carry out for inpatients. Furthermore, different patients would have different duration of thrombocytopenia, and some might remain in the hospital for other reasons after they were no longer thrombocytopenic. The decision was made to start observations for bleeding on the date of randomization, and continue until the first of the following events occurred: the subject died, was discharged alive from the hospital, was no longer thrombocytopenic, or had been studied for 30 days after the first platelet transfusion while on study.

> **EXAMPLE 1 (Continued)**
>
> **MAGIC:** All-cause mortality data can be collected by attempting to follow up with each study subject and/or his or her family, by searching medical records, by searching the National Death Index (in the United States) and similar databases, or by a combination of these techniques. The MAGIC study included a search of the medical record, and if necessary a follow-up phone call at 30 days, to determine the vital status of each subject or the date of death.

> **EXAMPLE 2 (Continued)**
>
> **PLADO:** A study of bleeding in thrombocytopenic patients could involve study staff assigning a bleeding grade for each patient-day, based on the bleeding scale the study has decided to use. Another option involves collection of the "raw" data necessary to determine a bleeding grade for each patient-day, with a computer algorithm to calculate the bleeding grade from the more detailed data. In either case, the "raw" data used by the study staff or the computer algorithm could be based only on chart review, or also on physical assessment and interview of the subject. The PLADO study decided to have study staff do daily physical assessments and interviews as well as chart reviews, because some instances of bleeding, especially more minor types of bleeding, may not always be noted in the medical chart as part of standard practice. The "raw" data were reported on case report forms, and a computer algorithm was used to determine the bleeding grades, to ensure uniformity in the assignment of grades.

make the definition more comparable between different study investigators, different study sites, or even different health care systems. Increasing comparability is often important. Some options may provide more detailed data for further analyses, which may be useful or may result in the costly collection of unnecessary data. The burden to subjects, study staff, and study finances should be considered as well.

Study Population
Another issue in trial design is selecting the population to be studied.

Careful consideration should be given to how broadly or narrowly to define the group of subjects to be studied (Fig. 2.2). A broadly defined study population will have a larger pool of eligible subjects. The screening phase of the study will be simpler, with lower labor costs and perhaps

Narrower eligibility criteria

- Less variability between subjects
- More easily interpretable results
- Reduced sample size (often)
- May be population of scientific interest

Broader eligibility criteria

- Larger pool of eligible subjects
- Simpler, lower-cost screening phase
- Higher enrollment rate
- May be more generalizable to actual clinical practice

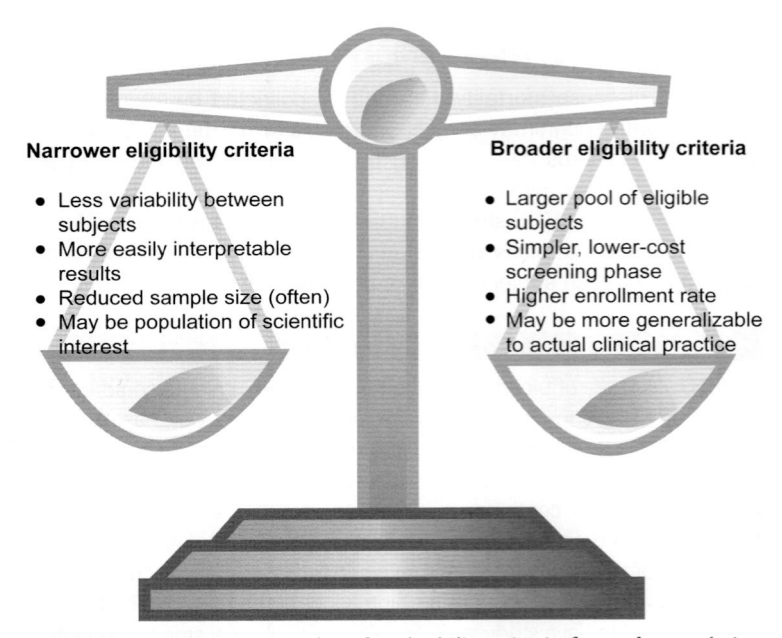

FIGURE 2.2 Narrower versus broader eligibility criteria for study population.

reduced costs for laboratory tests, imaging tests, and detailed chart reviews. Both of these aspects can lead to higher enrollment rates and thus faster completion of the study. In addition, the results of a study with fairly broad entry criteria may be more applicable to actual clinical practice than a study in which almost all patients seen in clinical practice were excluded from the study.

On the other hand, a more narrowly defined study population can also have advantages. There will be less variability between subjects, so the results of the study will be easier to interpret. Because there will be less "noise" in the data, it is possible that the sample size needed for the study may be decreased. And the narrower population may be the one of clinical interest (for example, patients with more severe, as opposed to very mild, levels of disease).

In addition to balancing these general considerations regarding how broadly the study population should be defined, here are other aspects that may apply to particular studies.

- Severity of disease (for treatment studies).
    Very mild disease may have little room for improvement, and treatment risks may outweigh potential benefits.

Very severe disease may be beyond the stage where the treatment could be expected to have an effect.
- Risk of disease (for prevention studies). Particular risk factor? High risk for one or more reasons? Population at large?
- Comorbidities that may make study results hard to interpret (e.g., end-stage cancer, for a study of treatment for MI that has all-cause 30-day mortality as the outcome).
- Treatment considerations.
    Are there subjects who are not good candidates for one or more treatment strategies in the study (e.g., tumor in an inoperable location)?
    Are there subjects who are at unacceptable risk for treatment side effects (e.g., allergic to a particular drug, or with impaired kidney function for a drug cleared by the kidneys)?
    Are there concomitant medications that cannot be taken in combination with one or more of the study treatments?
- Inpatient, outpatient, or both?

Unit of Treatment and Unit of Analysis: Choosing What to Randomize

In many clinical studies, the individual subject is the unit of both treatment and analysis. However, this is not always the case.

For example, an intervention may occur at the level of a school, a company, a hospital, or even a city. For example, hospitals might be randomized to use different types of hand sanitizers. The unit of analysis may still be the individual (each patient did or did not contract an infection while in the hospital), but in this situation the analysis will have to take into account that the treatment was assigned and applied to clusters of people, not to single individuals. (See the Cluster Design section in this chapter, as well as Chapter 4.)

For some studies, the unit of treatment and analysis may be smaller than an individual person. For example, two types of eyedrops could be compared in subjects with dry eyes, where the randomization determines whether the left eye gets treatment A and the right eye gets treatment B, or vice versa. Again, the analysis will need to take into account which eyes belong to the same person!

Superiority, Noninferiority, and Equivalence Trials: What is the Real Question?

The goal for many clinical studies is to determine whether two (or more) treatment strategies have different effects. For example, a study may be designed to show that a new treatment is better than no treatment or placebo, or better than an existing treatment. For these *superiority studies*, the null hypothesis is that there is no difference between treatment strategies. *The goal of a superiority study is to show, beyond a reasonable doubt, that there actually is a difference.*

However, some studies have different goals. *The goal of a **noninferiority study** is to show that an experimental treatment strategy is no worse than a standard treatment strategy.* Examples include:

- Studies to show no treatment is needed, when the commonly used treatment is not supported by good clinical data.
- Studies to show that minimal treatment is no less effective than intensive treatment.
- Studies to show that a new treatment with known advantages (safer, cheaper, easier to administer) is no less effective than a proven treatment.

For a noninferiority study, the researcher chooses a value, Δ, that is the minimum clinically significant difference between treatments. If high values of the outcome are bad (proportion of subjects with a bad result, high blood pressure values in hypertensive subjects), the null hypothesis is that the true proportion or mean in the experimental group is at least Δ higher than in the standard treatment group. The goal is to show, beyond a reasonable doubt, that the experimental treatment is not that much worse than the standard treatment. If it is much better, fine. If it is the same, or even a tiny bit worse, that is fine, too. All that is of interest is whether the data show it is very unlikely that the true difference is Δ or larger in the wrong direction.

*The goal of an **equivalence study** is to show that two treatment strategies have very similar effects.* Again, the researcher chooses a value Δ that is the minimum clinically significant difference between treatments. The null hypothesis is that the treatments differ by more than Δ *in either direction*. The goal is to show beyond a reasonable doubt that the absolute value of the true difference is less than Δ.

Figure 2.3 shows some examples of results that could occur in an equivalence study with an equivalence limit $\Delta = 1.2$. Each line in the figure indicates the point estimate and 90% confidence interval for the difference between the two treatment groups, from a simulated study where the true difference between the groups was 0.2. In studies 1, 8, and 9 we would not be able to declare equivalence, because the confidence interval extends beyond one or the other limit of equivalence. In the other studies, we would be able to declare equivalence.

There are some special considerations in designing a noninferiority study or an equivalence study, when the active control treatment has

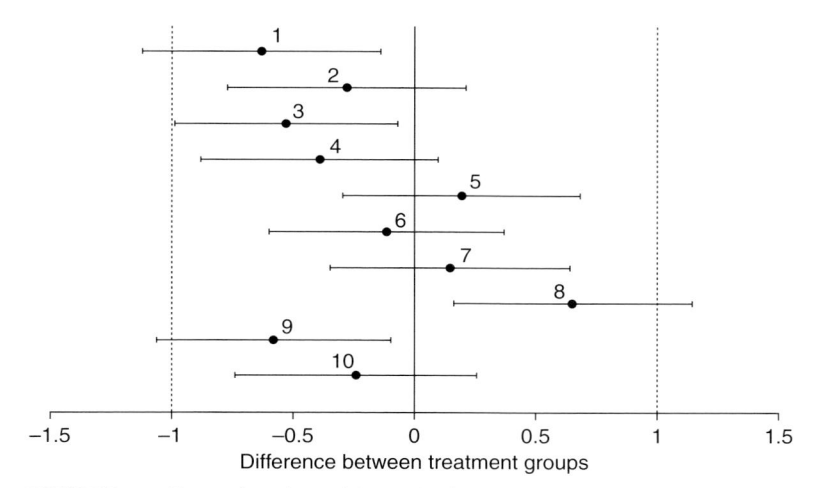

FIGURE 2.3 Examples of possible results for an equivalence trial.

been shown to be efficacious. As an example, suppose a prior, superiority, study showed that drug X reduced systolic blood pressure an average of 10 mm Hg more than placebo in a particular type of hypertensive patient, with 95% confidence interval 2 mm Hg to 18 mm Hg. We now want to show that a new experimental treatment, drug Y, is noninferior to drug X.

- The value of Δ should be small enough that drug Y would still be more effective than placebo if it was no more than Δ worse than drug X. A value of 8 for Δ would not be appropriate.
- The patient population for the noninferiority study should be similar to the patient population used to test drug X versus placebo. If we do not know that drug X is better than placebo in a given population, showing Y is noninferior to X does not provide much useful information.
- The other aspects of study design (when and how the outcome is measured) should also be similar to the previous study.

Because protocol violations, crossovers, and other problems with protocol compliance often make treatment groups look more similar to each other than they really are, excellent adherence to the protocol is even more important for noninferiority and equivalence studies than for superiority studies.

BLINDING: CONCEALING STUDY TREATMENTS FROM SUBJECTS AND INVESTIGATORS

Blinding or masking means concealing which treatment is being given. A single-blind study means that one party does not know what treatment is being given. Usually the study subject is the one who does not know the treatment, but sometimes the blinded party is the person or panel who will assess the subject's condition. A double-blind study means that neither the study subject, nor the clinical staff and assessors, know what treatment is being given.

The more subjective the study outcome is, the more important blinding will be to the validity of the study results. For example, if the study outcome is all-cause mortality, or the results of a platelet count taken 1 week after treatment begins, no subjectivity is involved. At the other extreme, if the study outcome is level of perceived pain, or quality of life, expectations and perceptions may vary depending on whether the subject believes an active treatment was given. In these cases blinding may be more important.

Even in studies with very objective outcomes, blinding may still be useful. For example, it may make it more difficult for study staff to guess which treatment is more likely to be assigned to the next enrolled subject, reducing bias in which subjects they enroll or when they decide to enroll a particular subject. For example, suppose Dr. Doe believes that the experimental treatment will turn out to be especially valuable for high-risk patients, but may not have much effect for low-risk patients. One day, Dr. Doe's study coordinator notifies him that two eligible subjects have just been admitted to the hospital: Mr. Smith, a low-risk patient, and Mrs. Jones, a high-risk patient. If Dr. Doe knows (or can make a good guess) that the next randomized subject will be assigned the experimental treatment, he may decide (consciously or not) to discuss the study with Mrs. Jones first, and be especially persuasive. This can lead to bias, because high-risk patients might tend to be assigned to the active treatment arm more often than they would be by chance alone.

Certain types of treatment may be difficult to blind. If an active treatment has common and noticeable side effects—either clinically apparent or measured by routine assays or procedures—true blinding may not be possible. For example, some cancer treatments may cause nausea or vomiting in a large percentage of subjects who receive them. As another example, if a study is comparing surgical treatment versus medication, blinding would involve sham surgery as well as placebo medication.

While the placebo medication may be easily implemented, sham surgery leads to logistic, ethical, and scientific questions. Will it be possible to involve a surgical team and facilities for sham surgery? Are the risks of giving anesthesia, without the possible benefit of the surgery, warranted? If the anesthesia itself may have an effect on the study outcome, will the results in the two treatment groups be more similar than they would be in "real life," where treatment by medication would not also involve sham surgery? As a general rule, sham operations are unethical.

GENERAL TYPES OF TRIAL DESIGN

Once the research question has been carefully specified, a choice must be made between various general types of trial design. Some studies will have a nonrandomized design. Advantages and disadvantages of nonrandomized designs are discussed in Chapter 3. In this section, the emphasis will be on randomized designs. The most common types are parallel group, factorial, crossover, and cluster.

Parallel Group Design: The Most Common Design

In a parallel group trial, each subject is randomized to a single treatment strategy (Fig. 2.4). The two (or more) groups of subjects are then followed in parallel to determine study outcomes. For example, patients with chronic arthritis pain could be randomized to one of two analgesic medications, A or B. As another example, a weight loss study could assign subjects to follow one of three exercise plans (swimming, walking, or running).

Usually a parallel group design will be the easiest design to implement, analyze, and interpret.

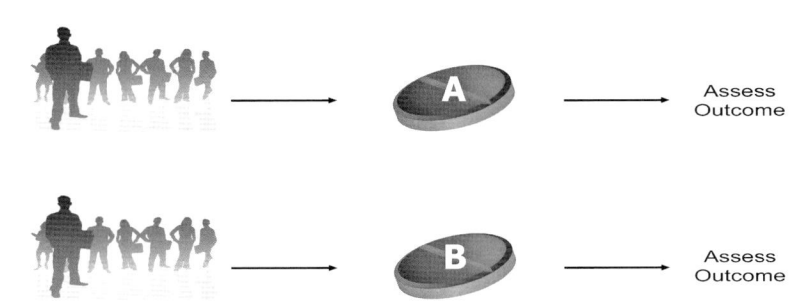

FIGURE 2.4 Parallel group design.

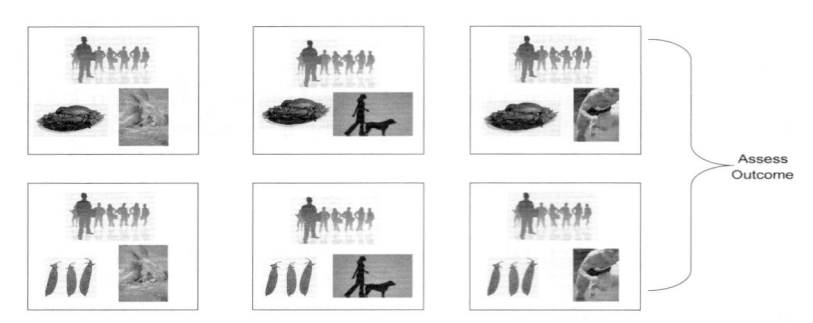

FIGURE 2.5 Factorial design.

Factorial Design: Studying Combinations of Treatments Within a Single Trial

Factorial designs are used to study the effects of two or more treatments, alone and in combination, within the same clinical trial (Fig. 2.5). For example, a weight loss study could investigate three different exercise plans (swimming, walking, or running) and two different dietary plans (high protein and vegetarian). In a complete factorial design, subjects would be randomized to each of the six (3 × 2) possible combinations of exercise and diet, and followed for study outcomes.

In a sense, a factorial design is a special case of a parallel group study, but the analysis and interpretation will be different. The goal is to separately estimate the effects of each treatment factor alone, and any interactive effects it has with the other treatment factors. In our example, at the end of the study the first step of analysis would be to see whether any differences in outcome between the three exercise plans were similar in diet group A and in diet group B, or whether the effect of the exercise plans differed depending on which diet was being followed. If there was no difference, the overall effects of the exercise plans can be compared to each other, including subjects from both diet plans, and the overall effects of the diet plans can be compared to each other, including subjects from all three exercise plans.

Crossover Design: Using Subjects as Their Own Controls

In a crossover design, each subject is assigned to more than one of the treatments being studied (Fig. 2.6) What is randomized is not which treatment each subject receives, but the order in which each subject receives the treatments. In between the treatment periods, there is often

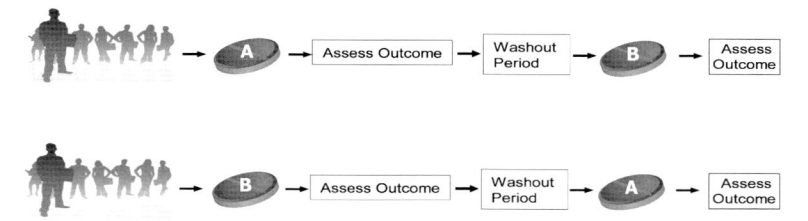

FIGURE 2.6 Crossover design.

a period of no treatment, to let any effects of the earlier treatment wear off before the next treatment begins. For example, patients with chronic arthritis pain could receive one analgesic medication for a month, take a week off analgesics to let the effects wear off, and then receive the other analgesic for a month.

The advantage of a crossover design is that each subject serves as his or her own control. This can reduce extraneous influences on the study outcome, and reduce the necessary sample size. For example, some subjects may tend to report higher levels of pain than other subjects with the same amount of inflammation, but this should be the case at both time periods.

However, crossover designs are only applicable to certain conditions, outcomes, and treatment strategies.

- The condition should be chronic, rather than acute. For example, a crossover placebo-controlled trial for pain after tooth extraction would not make sense. The pain may well have gone away before the second treatment begins, no matter whether the first treatment was the active medication or the placebo.
- Ideally, the condition being studied should be relatively stable within each individual subject, in the absence of treatment. If there are time trends, the analysis may help sort out the treatment effects from the time effects, but time trends will make the analysis more complicated.
- The outcome cannot be a one-time event such as death or first MI.
- No treatment strategy should be expected to cure the condition, or there will be nothing left for the later treatment to do.
- The treatments should not be expected to have effects that continue long after the treatment has stopped—that is, the washout period should be fairly short.

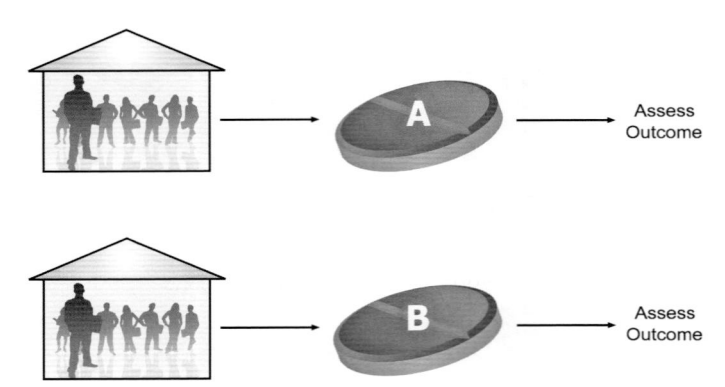

FIGURE 2.7 Cluster design.

Cluster Design: Randomizing Groups Instead of Individuals

In a cluster design (Fig. 2.7), whole groups of subjects are randomized, rather than individual subjects. Although outcomes may be measured at the individual level, **analysis and interpretation are accomplished at the cluster level,** because that is the unit of randomization.

Sometimes cluster randomization is used because the study intervention is by definition carried out at a group level. For example, suppose a study is investigating the usefulness of a media blitz of radio and TV public service announcements about the symptoms of heart attack and the importance of prompt treatment. By necessity, the intervention must be applied to large groups of subjects, such as cities. It is impossible to make sure the ad appears on the local news show seen by Mr. Smith but is not seen by Mrs. Jones who is watching the same show in the house next door!

Cluster randomization may also be used for reasons of feasibility. Suppose a study is comparing two different educational programs for training hospital staff how to reduce medication errors. Although it is theoretically possible to randomize individual staff members to receive one or the other educational program, it would be much easier and more cost-efficient to randomize entire hospitals to receive one or the other program. This approach is also more realistic in terms of how the more effective program would eventually be implemented.

Cluster randomization may also be used to reduce the chance of "cross-contamination" between treatments. In the example comparing educational programs, if individual staff members at the same hospital received different training sessions, they might discuss what they had learned with staff members assigned to the other program, making the effects of the two programs more similar than they really are.

If a cluster design is used, the analysis of study results must take into account which subjects were part of the same cluster (for example, which citizens were in the same city, or which patients were in the same hospital). Often subjects within a cluster will tend to be more similar to each other than they are to subjects in other clusters, so that it would be incorrect to assume their responses are independent. There may be additional differences between clusters at the cluster level as well (e.g., the number of medication orders the hospital pharmacy fills each day). These issues need to be addressed in the analysis plan.

ALLOCATION STRATEGIES

Most clinical studies are designed so that the number of subjects assigned to each treatment group is approximately the same. This usually will be the most statistically efficient allocation strategy. For example, suppose a study is being designed to have a 5% Type I error rate and 90% power to detect a treatment difference, assuming the control group has 30% mortality and the experimental group has 20% mortality. If allocation is equal between the two groups, 824 subjects will be needed, 412 in each group. If allocation is in a 2:1 ratio between the experimental and control groups, the study will need 918 subjects, 612 in the experimental group and 306 in the control group.

Sometimes there are good reasons to design a study with an allocation ratio other than 1:1. If there is a lot of information in the literature about how well the control treatment works in a given patient population, the investigators may decide to get more data about the experimental treatment by using a different allocation ratio, weighted more heavily to the experimental treatment. In the above example, a study using a 2:1 ratio results in approximately 50% more data about the experimental group, compared to a study using a 1:1 ratio (612 experimental group subjects rather than 412). However, this is at the expense of a total sample size that is more than 10% larger.

Another motivation for unequal allocation occurs when a new experimental device is being tested in a Phase II/III randomized trial, and each device has to be made individually, one after another. (Mass production usually is not implemented until the device has been proven effective.) This may severely limit the number of experimental devices available for the trial, especially if the device is complex. To ensure a feasible trial, more subjects may need to be assigned to the control group.[6]

Some studies do not use a fixed allocation ratio at all. One alternative is a "play the winner" approach. The initial allocation ratio may be 1:1, but as study data accumulate, the allocation ratio is changed so that subjects are more likely to be assigned to whichever treatment is doing better so far. Other studies may have an adaptive design that starts out with a 1:1 ratio, but at a predefined interim monitoring point may switch to a different ratio.

REFERENCES

1. MAGIC Steering Committee. Rationale and design of the magnesium in coronaries (MAGIC) study: a clinical trial to reevaluate the efficacy of early administration of magnesium in acute myocardial infarction. *Am Heart J.* 2000;139:10–14.
2. Magnesium in Coronaries (MAGIC) trial investigators. Early administration of intravenous magnesium to high-risk patients with acute myocardial infarction in the Magnesium in Coronaries (MAGIC) trial: a randomized controlled trial. *Lancet.* 2002;360:1189–1196.
3. CAST investigators. Preliminary report: effect of encainide and flecainide on mortality in a randomized trial of arrhythmia suppression after myocardial infarction. *N Engl J Med.* 1989;312:406–412.
4. Gmur J, Berger J, Schanz U, et al. Safety of stringent prophylactic platelet transfusion policy for patients with acute leukaemia. *Lancet.* 1991;338:1223–1226.
5. Heddle NM, Cook RJ, Webert KE, et al. Methodologic issues in the use of bleeding as an outcome in transfusion medicine studies. *Transfusion.* 2003;43:742–752.
6. Pennington DG, Griffith BP, McKinlay SM, et al. Evaluation of an implantable ventricular assist system for humans with chronic refractory heart failure: study overview. *ASAIO J.* 1995;41:11–15.

FURTHER READING

Cochran WG, Cox GM. *Experimental Designs.* New York: Wiley; 1950.
Fleiss JL. *The Design and Analysis of Clinical Experiments.* New York: Wiley; 1986.
Friedman LM, Furberg CD, DeMets DL. *Fundamentals of Clinical Trials.* 3rd ed. New York: Springer; 1998.
Heddle NM. The research question. *Transfusion.* 2007;47:15–17.
Piantadosi S. *Clinical Trials: A Methodologic Perspective.* New York: Wiley; 1997.
Senn S. *Statistical Issues in Drug Development.* New York: Wiley; 1997.
Snedecor GW, Cochran WG. *Statistical Methods.* 8th ed. Iowa University Press; 1989.
Tinmouth A, Hebert H. Interventional trials: an overview of design alternatives. *Transfusion.* 2007;47:565–567.

CHAPTER 3

Randomization: What It Is and How to Do It

CATHERINE E. HEWITT • DAVID J. TORGERSON

WHY IS RANDOMIZATION IMPORTANT?

There has been increased awareness of the need for basing health care decisions on the best available evidence.[1] Evidence of the effectiveness of an intervention is often sought using a variety of different research designs. Different research designs vary in their propensity for minimizing bias and the validity of their results. Bias of a particular study design can be thought of as the amount a study is likely to under- or overestimate the "true" effectiveness of the intervention under study,[2] while validity is confidence in the results from the study (internal validity) or confidence that the study findings can be generalized to the larger population (external validity).

Clinical research can broadly be split into two types: observational (Fig. 3.1) or experimental (Fig. 3.2).[3]

Within observational studies, the researcher does not have control over who gets the intervention, and effectiveness is established by comparing those who were naturally exposed to the intervention or treatment with those who were not exposed. Unfortunately, virtually all observational studies have a potential for bias because the groups formed naturally are unlikely to be comparable in terms of known and unknown characteristics.[4] Because group formation in an observational study is not a random process, it is possible, indeed likely, that group membership will be correlated with outcome ("case" or "not case" in the figures). For instance, people who receive a treatment from their doctor usually do so because they have been diagnosed with an illness. As these people have been "selected" into a treatment group, comparing them with an untreated control group is unlikely to be a fair test of the intervention. Consequently, random allocation is the best process for ensuring that

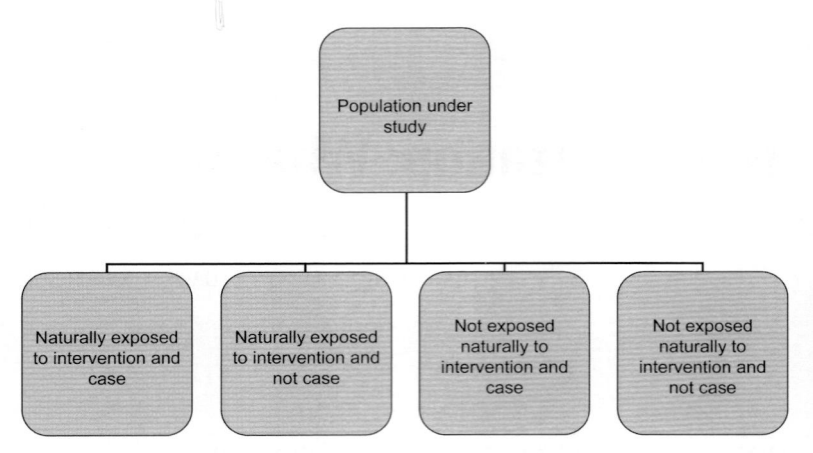

FIGURE 3.1 Example of an observational study.

selection bias is removed and there is a fair comparison between the treatment and control groups. In randomized controlled trials the researcher controls which participant gets which intervention.

The only nonrandomized study that, theoretically, is bias free is the regression discontinuity design.[5] This approach is rarely used in health care and consequently we do not discuss it further here.

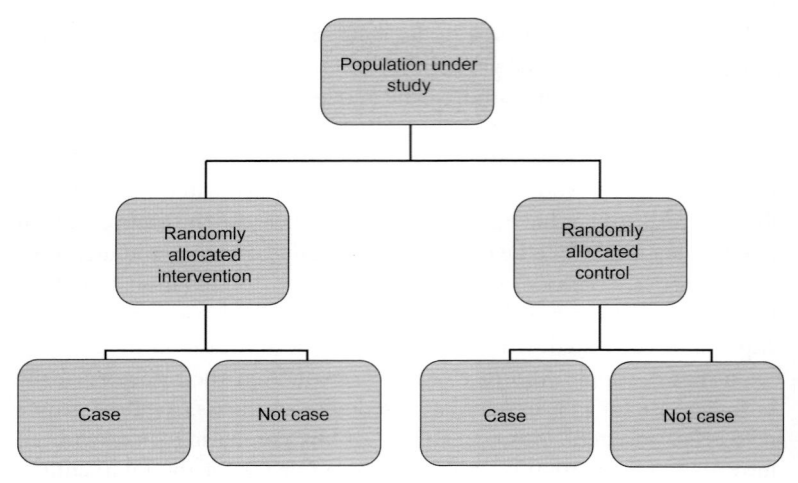

FIGURE 3.2 Example of an experimental study.

A randomized controlled trial in which the randomization process is truly random, is considered to be the most rigorous approach to establishing whether an intervention works. It provides the most reliable evidence because participants are randomly allocated, to be exposed to the intervention(s) under study by the play of chance. The main advantage of randomization is that it removes the potential for bias in the allocation of patients to different interventions, and the groups formed at baseline are generally balanced on known and unknown covariates.[6] Thus, selection bias should be avoided.

WHAT IS RANDOMIZATION?

Randomization is the process of allocating trial participants to study groups in which the probability of allocation can be calculated.[7] Secure randomization entails generating an unpredictable sequence for allocating participants to treatment groups, in a way that prevents foreknowledge of treatment assignment.[8] In practice, many haphazard or alternate assignment procedures masquerade as being random allocation.[3] Assignment procedures such as those based on birth date or zip code cannot be substituted as random, as the probability of random assignment is unknown and cannot be determined. Furthermore, haphazard assignment procedures have unknown statistical properties, whereas with random procedures the properties are known.[7] Another reason for randomizing is that statistical theory is based on the assumption of random sampling, and thus the use of randomization provides a basis for statistical inference.[9]

DIFFERENT METHODS OF RANDOMIZATION

Simple Randomization

The most straightforward way to allocate participants to treatment groups in a randomized controlled trial that still ensures population equality is to use simple (unrestricted) randomization. Simple randomization has been described as "elementary yet elegant."[10] A single randomization sequence is generated, and the next treatment in the list is allocated to the next participant who enters the trial. Because participants are usually recruited sequentially into the trial, we could also construct a sequence as we go along by randomly assigning each participant as he or she is recruited.

A drawback of using simple randomization is that by chance numerical and/or covariate imbalances can occur at baseline between trial arms. Numerical imbalances arise when, by chance, unequal numbers of participants are allocated to the treatment groups. Covariate imbalances arise when, by chance, there is an unequal distribution of participants with a particular covariate or variable that affects treatment outcomes between the trial arms. If a chance covariate imbalance is observed during the trial, then the imbalance needs to be adjusted in the analysis; otherwise it may result in a biased trial. Covariate imbalances are unimportant, in terms of having an effect on the overall result of the trial, if the variable has a weak or nonexistent relationship with treatment and outcome.[11] For example, gender may have little or no relationship with outcome; therefore an imbalance in the proportion of men and women within a trial would be of little importance. However, if by chance the groups differ at baseline on one or more confounding variables and the confounders are not treated as covariates in the analysis, then the trial result may be misleading. This effect could be in either direction (i.e., showing a positive result when really a negative result is true, or vice versa). Restricted randomization methods are often employed to reduce the likelihood of such events.[12]

Restricted Randomization

If chance numerical imbalances do arise between groups, then there may be a cosmetic concern; however, the main issue is that the power of a statistical test is reduced.[13] Conventionally, trials are designed with a power of 80%.[3] A power of 80% implies that if the trial were conducted many times, then 80% of these trials would find a statistically significant difference between two treatments if a real difference of the specified magnitude exists in the population. If a numerical imbalance of 0.7 occurred (that is, 70% are allocated to one group and 30% to the other), then the subsequent power of the statistical test would be reduced to 73%. Consequently to maximize statistical power it is usually the case that the group sizes should be as similar as possible. However, the threat of numerical imbalance to a study's power is only relevant when sample sizes are small (e.g., < 50 participants). For larger studies, then, the probability of having significant numerical imbalances declines with increasing sample size. Thus, trials with a sample size of 50 or above using simple randomization have less than 0.005 probability of a numerical imbalance as high as 0.7.

Another reason that sometimes justifies the use of restricted randomization is to ensure balance upon some known, and measurable, covariate. We can ensure, for example, through using restricted randomization techniques, that exact balance can be achieved in age or other important predictors of outcome using stratified randomization. Combining stratified randomization with some form of analysis of covariance can improve the power of our study *if the sample size is small.* As the sample size increases, the prevalence of the prognostic factor becomes less important in terms of the subsequent possibility of an imbalance arising. For example, in a trial with an overall sample size of 100, there is a less than 0.01 probability that there will be a chance baseline covariate imbalance that would reduce the relative efficiency below 0.9. In addition, for an overall sample size of 50, there is a less than 0.01 probability that there will be a chance baseline covariate imbalance that would reduce the relative efficiency below 0.85. For trials with 50 participants or fewer, there are small gains in statistical efficiency when stratified randomization (with a stratified analysis) is used instead of simple randomization (with a stratified analysis).

Variability in workload between the treatments under study is probably a more important reason why trialists would want to ensure balance between trial arms. If the treatments under study vary in the amount of time required to undertake or implement them, then having more participants allocated to one of the trial arms may cause delays in the treatment of participants. It is important to try to reduce the amount of time between recruitment and when the participant actually receives treatment. One example of needing to ensure equity in workload was in a trial examining how improved attention to nutritional status and dietary intake affected postoperative clinical outcomes among elderly women with hip fracture.[14] Participants were randomized either to receive the conventional pattern of nurse- and dietician-led care or to receive the additional personal attention of dietetic assistants. The dietetic assistants could only manage a certain number of participants per day; hence if a large number of participants were by chance randomly allocated to the intervention arm, then the dietetic assistants would be unable to manage to treat the participants within the required timeframe. Conversely, if a large number of participants were by chance randomly allocated to the control arm, then the dietetic assistants would have little work to undertake for the trial. Thus, to ensure equity in the dietetic assistants' workload throughout the trial, restricted randomization was used.

Another reason for wanting to ensure balance is cost, which is especially of concern when more than one center is involved in the trial.[15] For example, if the experimental treatment is more expensive than the control treatment, and in one of the centers more participants are allocated to the experimental treatment, then this would lead to inequity in costs across centers.

Another situation that may arise is if one of the interventions has major resource planning implications, such as in a trial of a surgical intervention versus a medical management intervention.[16] In order to plan resources effectively, surgical slots would need to be pre-booked; sometimes this may need to be months in advance. If simple randomization was used, then by chance an excess of participants might be allocated to one of the trial arms. The consequences of this would either be an overload in the surgical arm with delays in the treatment of participants or wastage of pre-booked slots in surgery. Neither of these consequences is desirable, and may lead to further problems within the trial.

Finally, if recruitment is anticipated to be relatively small and is spread over a long period of time, then simple randomization could lead to bias in terms of temporal effects. For instance, if the trial was only recruiting a few participants a month, then it is possible that all or most participants recruited over the winter period might by chance be allocated to one of the groups. If season affected outcome, then this may introduce a seasonal bias.

Restricted randomization is more common than simple randomization. In a review of 150 randomized trials published in *Lancet* and the *New England Journal of Medicine* in 2001, researchers found that 47% (n = 71) of the trials reported using some form of restricted randomization[17]; while a more recent survey of 232 trials published in 2002 in four major medical journals found that only 9% used simple randomization.[18] Indeed, in this study we found a relationship between randomization method and total sample sizes with trials using simple randomization having the smallest median sample size, which is the opposite of what theory would predict.

HOW TO RANDOMIZE

Simple Randomization

Simple randomization sequences for allocating participants to treatment groups can be constructed in many ways—for example, by tossing a coin, throwing a die, or dealing preshuffled cards. Although these approaches do, in theory, represent random methods of allocating participants to treatment groups, they can easily become nonrandom in practice, because there is limited allocation concealment and the series can easily be altered. For instance, if an investigator tosses a coin to allocate participants to two intervention groups, and 19 heads and 20 tails have been thrown and the next toss is tails, then the investigator may be tempted to allocate the person to the heads group rather than the tails group. In addition, manual methods of generating the randomization sequences (e.g., tossing a coin, throwing a die, or dealing preshuffled cards) may be seen as less robust, because the sequence cannot be verified and repeating the process may lead to a different randomization sequence being generated.[10] Therefore, tables of random numbers,[19] or computer pseudo–random-number generators with a known seed, are preferable methods to produce simple randomization sequences.

In the following sections, three of the most frequently used methods of generating a restricted randomization sequence are discussed: block randomization, stratified randomization, and minimization.

Blocked Randomization

Block randomization is a commonly used form of restricted randomization.[10] In block randomization, the sequence is broken down into discrete blocks. As participants enter the trial, they are allocated to the next treatment in the block. Once the block is full, the next participant is allocated to the treatment in the next randomly selected block. This process is repeated until the required sample size is achieved. For example, if a constant block size of four were used, in a trial of two treatments (A and B) and there was an equal allocation ratio, then there would be six possible ways of arranging the two treatments within the blocks (Fig. 3.3).

These six blocks are then used to create the allocation sequence. The blocks could be randomly chosen, for example, by labeling the series of allocations above from one to six (AABB, ABAB, and so on), and then using a random numbers table to determine the order of the six possible ways of arranging the blocks. If a constant block size is used without stratification, then the number of participants in the two groups should only differ by a maximum of half the block size and hence the chance of numerical imbalance will be eliminated. For instance, if a block size of four is used without stratification, then the maximum numerical imbalance expected would be two. It is also possible to generate the randomization sequence using a mixture of block sizes or randomly selected block sizes from a given range. These approaches are often used to reduce prediction of randomization sequences. Nevertheless, if random block sizes are used and the investigator simply guesses that the next treatment allocation in the sequence will be the one that has occurred least often, then using random block sizes will not reduce predictability of the sequence.

| AABB | ABAB | BBAA | BABA | BAAB | ABBA |

FIGURE 3.3 Example of block randomization.

Stratified Randomization
When stratification is used, participants are divided into strata and restricted randomization sequences are generated for each stratum. For example, if the stratifying variable is presence or absence of diabetes, then two blocked randomization sequences will be needed: one for participants with diabetes and the second for participants without diabetes. The total number of strata is calculated by multiplying the number of levels of each factor. For the example, there would be two levels (people with diabetes and people without diabetes); however, if the randomization was also stratified on age (≤ 50 and > 50), then there would be four levels (people with diabetes and ≤ 50, people with diabetes and > 50, people without diabetes and ≤ 50, and people without diabetes and > 50). It is clear that as the number of stratifying variables increases, the number of randomization sequences needed also increases rapidly. Note that within a stratified variable, imbalance can only be half the block size.

Minimization
When stratification is used, as the number of stratifying variables increases so does the number of randomization sequences required to implement the procedure. This can lead to more strata than participants in the trial and/or increase the chance that various cells produced by the stratification will include no participants; this is especially true in small trials.[20] Hence minimization is often used to overcome this problem.

Minimization can be thought of as an extreme form of stratification. When minimization is used, the first few participants to be randomized are allocated using simple randomization. If an imbalance in the variables that are considered important arises, then the next participant is allocated to the group that minimizes the imbalance. The frequencies of the key prognostic variables in each of the treatment groups are monitored throughout the randomization process; this is generally undertaken using a computer. For example, in a trial of two treatments (A and B) with an equal allocation ratio, if group A has a higher average age and more participants with diabetes compared with group B, then the next older diabetic participant will be allocated to treatment group B to balance the groups on these two variables (Table 3.1). If the totals of the prognostic variables are sufficiently similar in the treatment groups, then simple randomization is used to allocate the next participant.

Minimization is a largely nonrandom method of sequence generation, as the characteristics are (wholly or partly) determining which group the participants are allocated to. Some researchers include a random element in the minimization algorithm by allocating only a randomly selected

Table 3.1 Example of Minimization Procedure

	Age (mean)	Diabetes (%)
Intervention A	70	50
Intervention B	65	40
Participant to be randomized	73	Diabetic
Allocation	Intervention B	

proportion (e.g., 80%) of the participants to the treatment group that minimizes the differences in the prognostic factors.[21] This method obviously leads to a reduction in the efficiency of balance achieved in the prognostic factors across the treatment groups; but this is still much higher than that achieved by simple randomization.[22]

Pairwise Randomization
One recently proposed method of randomization that could potentially be used to resolve the conflict between the desire to achieve balance and the need to reduce predictability, is pairwise randomization.[23] Pairwise randomization requires two participants to be randomized at the same time. One participant is randomly selected and the treatment is allocated by minimization (if there are important prognostic variables) or simple randomization (if there are no important prognostic variables); and then the other participant is nonrandomly allocated to the other trial arm. As both participants are equally likely to be randomly allocated to the trial arms (i.e., both participants have 50% chance of being selected to be randomly allocated), foreknowledge of treatment allocations is prevented.

The only potential drawback of using pairwise randomization to randomly allocate participants to trial arms would be if recruitment were slow. If pairwise randomization is used and recruitment is slow, then there may be a long time between recruiting a participant to the trial and the participant receiving his or her allocated treatment. This again highlights the tradeoffs that need to be made when choosing the optimum randomization method for the individual trial. Unfortunately, there is no single method of randomization that can be advocated to be used in all trials, and tradeoffs need to be made, especially in terms of balance and predictability. In those instances where small chance imbalances would be of little concern, then using simple randomization may be the preferred option. Nevertheless, if there are strong reasons to ensure balance, then using restricted randomization (e.g., pairwise randomization) may be necessary.

PROTECTING THE RANDOMIZATION SEQUENCE

Randomization, if conducted properly, will remove selection bias. However, as Archie Cochrane said:

> The RCT is a very beautiful technique, of wide applicability, but as with everything else there are snags.[24]

Although the RCT should, in theory, eliminate selection bias, unless additional steps are taken to preserve the initial randomization sequence, selection bias can be reintroduced. Unfortunately, history tells us that many researchers and clinicians will not keep to the random allocation procedure if they become aware of future allocations. For a variety of reasons, some people will select participants into a treatment arm, and if this is done, selection bias is introduced and the trial can no longer be considered a randomized controlled study. Therefore, it is important that trials use a secure method of randomization.

Randomization can be undermined if the allocation sequence is not concealed from the investigator(s) enrolling participants. This is because knowledge of the allocation sequence can sometimes influence the decision to recruit a participant, such that participants are "selected" into their treatment groups. In 1999, it was acknowledged that Bradford Hill's main motivation for advocating the randomized controlled trial in 1946, rather than quasi-random methods such as alternation, was to eliminate bias in the selection of participants.[25,26]

Unfortunately, allocation concealment does not prevent investigators guessing or predicting the next treatment allocation when previous treatment allocations are known. This situation is of greatest concern in open trials—that is, trials that do not or cannot use placebo control. In an open trial, a participant is enrolled and the allocated group is revealed to the participant and the investigator. The investigator can use this information to guess or predict future allocations with a greater degree of certainty if restricted forms of random allocation, such as blocked randomization, are used compared with simple randomization. Another example is if the covariates used in a minimization algorithm are known in advance; then there is the potential for the investigator to keep a running total of the covariates and predict with certainty all of the upcoming treatment allocations when an imbalance arises.[17]

Center is often used as a stratification variable in multicenter studies. Center can be incorporated into the randomization sequence when minimization is used in two ways: randomization sequences are stratified by center before using minimization or by including center in the minimization algorithm. Scott and McPherson[27] investigated numerical and covariate imbalances when the different minimization strategies were used in a multicenter trial.[27] Their results highlighted that when the randomization sequence was stratified by clinician, before using minimization, larger numerical and covariate imbalances were present compared to the other approaches.

The potential effect of selection bias is that wrong conclusions could be drawn about the beneficial or harmful effects of the treatment or intervention under study.[28] For example, if younger participants are diverted or self-selected into the treatment group, then the treatment effect may be overestimated. Conversely, if younger participants are preferentially allocated or self-selected into the control group, then the treatment effect may be underestimated. The presence of selection bias within an RCT invalidates the design and has potentially damaging consequences. If investigators are unaware, or fail to report, that their RCT has been compromised, then the worry is that the results are interpreted as being more reliable than an observational study, when in reality they are not.[29] Prevention of selection bias is one of the key reasons why randomization is used in practice.

Evidence for Subversion of Randomization

There are a number of published studies that suggest that randomization has been subverted and selection bias introduced. One study that has reported the intricate details of subversion was published in 1995 and used anonymous accounts from more than 20 epidemiology workshops for medical residents and medical school junior faculty.[30] Over an 8-year period, data were collected from between 400 and 500 people involved in the workshops, which were held to discuss allocation concealment. The participants were asked "how many of the participants had deciphered, or had witnessed someone else decipher, an assignment sequence?" After some initial apprehension, more than half of the participants relayed at least one instance of deciphering. The examples of subversion from the epidemiology workshops were all relating to situations where allocation sequences were public knowledge or the concealment of the allocation was inadequate, such as using sealed envelopes that can be tampered with.

Research investigating the effect of methodologic quality, which incorporates an analysis of adequacy of allocation concealment, does suggest an impact on effect sizes.[31–35] In 1995, Schulz et al. assessed the methodologic quality of 250 controlled trials from 33 meta-analyses from the Cochrane Pregnancy and Childbirth Database.[32] They found that trials in which concealment was classified as inadequate or unclear were associated with larger estimates of treatment effects by 30% to 40% compared with those classified as having adequate allocation concealment. A second review—this time investigating the efficacy of interventions used for circulatory and digestive diseases, mental health, and pregnancy and childbirth—included 11 randomly selected meta-analyses involving 127 RCTs.[34] The results indicate that in those clinical trials reporting inadequate rather than adequate allocation concealment, the estimate of treatment effects was 37% greater. Because allocation concealment can be achieved in virtually every individually randomized trial, sufficient steps should be taken in the design phase to ensure that this happens.

A relatively common method of allocation concealment is to use sealed opaque envelopes. In previous studies exploring the effects of allocation concealment, investigators classified sealed, opaque, and sequentially numbered envelopes as an adequate method of allocation concealment.[32] However, the envelope system may not be an adequate method of allocation concealment. For instance, if the person who recruits participants also opens the envelopes to allocate participants to the treatment groups, then the allocation list could be observed if the envelope is held against a bright light, such as those found in radiology departments[32]; or alternatively, the envelopes could be opened in advance.[36] Even if the envelopes are sequentially numbered, this cannot prevent the scheduling of participants but only reordering of the envelopes. Subversion of allocation using sealed opaque envelopes has been reported.[32,36,37]

A review has been undertaken to describe the current methods of allocation concealment adopted by trialists, and to investigate the prevalence of adequate concealment.[38] They focused on 234 trials published in four general medical journals (*British Medical Journal, Lancet, Journal of the American Medical Association*, and the *New England Journal of Medicine*) in 2002. Of the 234 trials included in the review, only 132 (56%) were classified as using adequate concealment and 118 (89%) of these used independent allocation. Independent allocation included allocation using a telephone, fax, or pager to a randomization service. Despite the importance of adequate allocation concealment being widely accepted by trial methodologists, a substantial proportion of trials recently published in major medical journals did not report adequate concealment methods.

Two potential examples of prediction from the literature are outlined next. The first potential example was in an open trial of rehabilitation care for patients after a hip fracture.[39] The investigator used block randomization and established a telephone allocation system in which nursing staff recruited participants. The block size was six, but this was constructed by putting two blocks of three together. Using two blocks of three meant that the third and last allocation could be perfectly predicted if the allocation sequence was recorded. Upon completion of recruitment and follow-up, the researcher noticed that frailer participants had been allocated preferentially to the intervention group. Further investigation of this imbalance revealed that part of the problem was in the third allocation of the block (i.e., one of those that could be perfectly predicted) and it happened only part of the time. It is unclear how the allocation was undermined.

The second example of this type of subversion was in a trial comparing tension-free vaginal tape with colposuspension as primary treatment for stress incontinence.[40] The article reported that participants were allocated to treatment groups using a computer-generated block randomization sequence of two lengths (four and six) via a telephone system. In a subsequent commentary, by one of the investigators, it was reported that the original randomization sequence was generated using a single block size of four.[41] It transpires that one of the individuals involved in the trial released the block size to one of the investigators. Because this was an open trial, the last allocation could always be perfectly predicted, and in some cases the last two allocations, if a record of previous treatment allocations was maintained. No details were given of the effects of releasing the block size, only that the block size was changed, and as this occurred early in the trial no significant bias was introduced.

A small exploratory study conducted by Brown et al. in 2005 focused on whether people involved in trials do try to predict treatment allocations, and if they do, how they predict treatment allocations.[15] Twenty-five clinicians and research nurses, who were at the time recruiting participants into studies being undertaken at the clinical trials research unit, were surveyed. They asked the participants the following questions:

1. Do you try to predict treatment allocations?
2. If so, is there a method/technique that you use to make predictions?
3. Does your prediction affect whether or not you enter a participant into a trial?
4. If you do not try to predict treatment allocation, what are your reasons for this?
5. Does your decision to predict treatment allocation depend upon the trial in question, and are there any other factors that contribute to your decision?

Surprisingly, 4 out of the 25 (16%) people questioned reported that they did try to predict forthcoming treatment allocations. All 4 of them reported using the same method to make their predictions; that is, they kept a log of all of the previous treatment allocations. Others were a little coy about whether or not they tried to predict treatment allocations by saying that they *hoped* some participants would be randomized to particular treatments. The reasons they gave for this hope were participant orientated; for example, it would be easier for the participants to travel to receive one of the treatments and that the clinicians and research nurses perceived particular treatments to be beneficial for certain participants. For the group of people who reportedly did not attempt to predict treatment allocations, the reasons why they did not fell into two groups. The first group of people did not attempt to predict upcoming allocations as they were aware of the importance of randomization and concealment. For example, they gave answers like "aware it was wrong" and "remain impartial to the treatments." The second group of people claimed to be unaware that treatment allocations could be predicted. They gave responses like "unable to, allocation is out of our hands"; and several were not aware that it was possible and were under the impression that doing so would be too complicated and therefore did not try.

It is also worth noting that if an individual is presented with an opportunity to undermine the randomization sequence, it does not mean that he or she will do so. This was highlighted in the survey just mentioned.[15] One respondent relayed an incidence where a distinct pattern had emerged in the treatment allocations and two participants were to be randomized at the same time. Instead of randomizing the participants themselves, they called upon another person to select the order in which the participants should be randomized to avoid any possible bias. Hence, given the opportunity, not everyone will subvert a trial. Nevertheless, it is important that the potential to undermine the randomization sequence is minimized to prevent the possibility of subversion arising.

CONCLUSION

For a simple process, there are a surprising number of ways of randomly allocating participants to treatment groups. This chapter has given a brief overview of some of the most common methods of allocation. There are other more rarely used approaches to randomization that we have not covered in this chapter. Indeed, it is possible to write a whole book about how to randomize (for example, see Rosenberger and Lachin[13]).

However, the key issue with respect to randomization is to preserve the random allocation process. Consequently, the choice of method should be principally determined by the need to avoid bias. In a perfect world, any of the approaches described in this chapter would satisfactorily avoid bias *if they were correctly implemented*. Unfortunately, this is not the case, and the researcher should always be aware of the potential for subversion of even the most elegant randomization schedule. For large trials that recruit participants at regular intervals and where there is little problem of scheduling treatment resources (e.g., pharmaceutical studies), we recommend the use of simple randomization with prespecified covariate adjustment rather than stratified allocation. The reason for this is that restricted allocation gives little additional benefit in terms of power but increases the risk of introducing selection bias through subversion. Of course the point needs to be reemphasized that simple randomization is only superior in its resistance to subversion compared with restricted allocation methods if the process is concealed from recruiting physicians and researchers.

Pairwise randomization is a useful alternative if simple randomization potentially leads to unwanted imbalances. If stratified randomization is needed, then avoiding using center as a stratification variable will reduce the risk of predictability and consequently subversion.

On the other hand, if the sample size is small and/or recruitment is likely to be slow, then a key challenge is to minimize the possibility of chance imbalances. If the researcher thinks that chance is more of a threat than subversion, then one of the restricted methods described earlier should be employed. Nevertheless, whichever method is used, it is essential to use a process that is secure and can yield a verifiable audit trail of the process.

REFERENCES

1. Evans D. Hierarchy of evidence: a framework for ranking evidence evaluating healthcare interventions. *J Clin Nurs*. 2003;12:77–84.
2. Altman DG, Bland JM. Statistics notes: how to randomise. *BMJ*. 1999; 319:703–704.
3. Schulz KF, Grimes DA. *The Lancet Handbook of Essential Concepts in Clinical Research*. Edinburgh: Elsevier; 2006.
4. Grimes DA, Schulz KF. Bias and causal associations in observational research. *Lancet*. 2002;359:248–252.
5. Torgerson DJ, Torgerson CJ. *Designing Randomised Controlled Trials in Health Education and the Social Sciences*. Basingstoke: Palgrave Macmillan; 2008.
6. May GS, Demets DL, Friedman LM, et al. The randomized clinical trial—bias in analysis. *Circulation*. 1981;64:669–673.

7. Blume J, Peipert JF. Randomization in controlled clinical trials: why the flip of a coin is so important. *J Am Assoc Gynecol Laparosc.* 2003;11:320–325.
8. Juni P, Altman DG, Egger M. Systematic reviews in health care: assessing the quality of controlled clinical trials. *BMJ.* 2001;323:42–46.
9. Young J. When should you use statistics? *Swiss Med Weekly.* 2005;135: 337–338.
10. Schulz KF, Grimes DA. Generation of allocation sequences in randomised trials: chance, not choice. *Lancet.* 2002;359:515–519.
11. Altman DG. Comparability of randomised groups. *Statistician.* 1985;34: 125–136.
12. Lachin JM. Statistical properties of randomization in clinical trials. *Controlled Clin Trials.* 1988;9:289–311.
13. Rosenberger W, Lachin J. *Randomization in Clinical Trials: Theory and Practice.* New York: Wiley; 2002.
14. Duncan DG, Beck SJ, Hood K, et al. Using dietetic assistants to improve the outcome of hip fracture: a randomised controlled trial of nutritional support in an acute trauma ward. *Age Ageing.* 2006;35:148–153.
15. Brown S, Thorpe H, Hawkins K, et al. Minimization-reducing predictability for multi-centre trials whilst retaining balance within centre. *Stat Med.* 2005;24:3715–3727.
16. PDSURG trial. Available from: http://www.pdsurg.bham.ac.uk/trial/.
17. Scott NW, McPherson GC, Ramsay CR, et al. The method of minimization for allocation to clinical trials: a review. *Controlled Clin Trials.* 2002;23: 662–674.
18. Hewitt CE, Torgerson DJ. Is restricted randomisation necessary? *BMJ.* 2006;332:1506–1508.
19. Rich M. *A Million Random Digits with 100,000 Normal Deviates.* Santa Monica: RAND; 2001.
20. Hagino A, Hamada C, Yoshimura I, et al. Statistical comparison of random allocation methods in cancer clinical trials. *Controlled Clin Trials.* 2004;25:572–584.
21. Pocock SJ, Simon R. Sequential treatment assignment with balancing for prognostic factors in controlled clinical trial. *Biometrics.* 1975;31:103–115.
22. Altman DG, Bland JM. Treatment allocation by minimization. *BMJ.* 2005;330:843.
23. Daniels J, Wheatley K, Gray R. Pairwise randomisation to balance within centres without possible foreknowledge of allocation. *Controlled Clin Trials.* 2003;24:104–105.
24. Cochrane A. *Effectiveness and Efficiency: Random Reflections on Health Services.* London: Nuffield Provincial Hospitals Trust; 1972.
25. Chalmers I. Why transition from alternation to randomisation in clinical trials was made. *BMJ.* 1999;319:1372.
26. Chalmers I. Comparing like with like: some historical milestones in the evolution of methods to create unbiased comparison groups in therapeutic experiments. *Int J Epidemiol.* 2001;30:1156–1164.

27. Scott N, McPherson G. Minimization in multicentre clinical trials. *Controlled Clin Trials.* 2003;24:175S–175S.
28. Gluud LL. Bias in clinical intervention research. *Am J Epidemiol.* 2006;163: 493–501.
29. Torgerson DJ, Torgerson CJ. Avoiding bias in randomised controlled trials in educational research. *Br J Educ Studies.* 2003;51:36–45.
30. Schulz KF. Subverting randomization in controlled trials. *JAMA.* 1995;274:1456–1458.
31. Emerson JD, Burdick E, Hoaglin DC, et al. An empirical study of the possible relation of treatment differences to quality scores in controlled randomized clinical trials. *Controlled Clin Trials.* 1990;11:339–352.
32. Schulz KF, Chalmers I, Hayes RJ, et al. Empirical evidence of bias: Dimensions of methodological quality associated with estimates of treatment effects in controlled trials. *JAMA.* 1995;273:408–412.
33. Chalmers T, Celano P, Sacks H, et al. Bias in treatment assignment in controlled clinical trials. *N Engl J Med.* 1983;309:1358–1361.
34. Moher D, Pham B, Jones A, et al. Does quality of reports of randomised trials affect estimates of intervention efficacy reported in meta-analyses? *Lancet.* 1998;352:609–613.
35. Kjaergard LL, Villumsen J, Gluud C. Reported methodologic quality and discrepancies between large and small randomized trials in meta-analyses. *Ann Int Med.* 2001;135:982–989.
36. Kennedy A, Grant A. Subversion of allocation in a randomised controlled trial. *Controlled Clin Trials.* 1997;18:S77–S78.
37. Swingler GH, Zwarenstein M. An effectiveness trial of a diagnostic test in a busy outpatients department in a developing country: issues around allocation concealment and envelope randomization. *J Clin Epidemiol.* 2000;53:702–706.
38. Hewitt C, Hahn S, Torgerson DJ, et al. Adequacy and reporting of allocation concealment: review of recent trials published in four general medical journals. *BMJ.* 2005;330:1057–1058.
39. Turner J. Randomised trial of a high dependency unit: a cautionary tale. PhD thesis. *Health Sciences.* York: University of York; 2002.
40. Ward K, Hilton P. Prospective multicentre randomised trial of tension-free vaginal tape and colposuspension as primary treatment for stress incontinence. *BMJ.* 2002;325:67–70.
41. Hilton P. Trials of surgery for stress incontinence—thoughts on the "Humpty Dumpty principle." *Br J Obstet Gynaecol.* 2002;109:1081–1088.

FURTHER READING

Brown S, Thorpe H, Hawkins K, et al. Minimization-reducing predictability for multi-centre trials whilst retaining balance within centre. *Stat Med.* 2005;24:3715–3727.

Chalmers I. Why transition from alternation to randomization in clinical trials was made. *BMJ*. 1999;319:1372.

Cochrane A. *Effectiveness and Efficiency: Random Reflections on Health Services*. London: Nuffield Provincial Hospitals Trust; 1972.

Hewitt C, Hahn S, Torgerson DJ, et al. Adequacy and reporting of allocation concealment: review of recent trials published in four general medical journals. *BMJ*. 2005:330;1057–1058.

Lachin JM. Statistical properties of randomization in clinical trials. *Controlled Clin Trials*. 1988;9:289–311.

CHAPTER 4

Setting Sample Size for Randomized Clinical Trials

XIN TIAN • SONJA M. MCKINLAY • NANCY L. GELLER

Planning a randomized controlled trial (RCT) requires carefully estimating the sample size needed to definitively answer the question posed. The first step is to state a clear hypothesis. For RCTs comparing two treatments or an active treatment to a placebo, the hypothesis is usually that there is no difference between the treatments under study. This is termed a null hypothesis (usually denoted as H_0), and is "rejected" when the conclusion of the trial is that one or the other treatment is superior. When the null hypothesis is not rejected, the evidence is not convincing that there is a difference in treatment effect.

Perhaps the most important aspect of designing a trial is calculating the sample size—the total number of subjects required across all treatment groups (for example, if there are three treatment groups, then the total sample size is the sum of the number in each of the three groups). This number is the major determinant of how long the trial will take (trial duration = accrual period + follow-up); how many sites will be needed to accrue the total subjects in a reasonable time frame (accrual period); and how much the trial will cost.

The equations used to estimate sample size make use of a number of variables that must be supplied. This chapter discusses what must be considered when setting sample size; actual formulas can be found in the references. Understanding what is needed for sample size estimation is critical because the trialist must supply these parameters, or at least estimates of them, to the statistician actually making the calculation of sample size. These parameters include:

- *Significance level*. The probability that a null hypothesis that is true will be rejected (the Type I error).

- *Power.* The probability that the trial will detect a real difference if one actually exists (1 − Type II error).
- *Primary endpoint of the trial.* The outcome variable specified for use in the power calculations, which is generally the endpoint of greatest interest.
- *Types of endpoints.* Endpoints can be dichotomous ("yes or no"), continuous (any value within some range), censored (endpoint may not yet have occurred when the end of the follow-up is reached), or composite (comprising more than one event).
- *Effect size.* The minimum difference in treatment effect that would be clinically relevant.
- *Treatment group strategies.* This includes choice of control group as well as experimental group(s) to maximize the effect size.
- *Subject accrual.* In general, the more sites and fewer exclusion criteria, the faster accrual will be.
- *Trial duration.* The longer the follow-up, the greater the number of events and thus the smaller the sample size (all else being the same).
- *Dilution.* When the randomized treatment is not given or completed, for a variety of reasons, and instead another treatment or no treatment is given, the treatment effect may become smaller.
- *Interim looks for efficacy.* Many studies have an interim monitoring plan. A Data and Safety Monitoring Board views results by treatment group at intervals during the study, and if there is overwhelming evidence that one treatment is better than the other, according to prespecified boundaries, the study may be stopped early. However, to preserve Type I error, the sample size must be increased slightly to account for the extra looks at the data.

The next section encompasses brief discussions of all the key ingredients that result in an optimal sample size. This is followed, in the next two sections, with how these ingredients are used for superiority trials, then for equivalence and noninferiority trials. The following section touches on different approaches for complex designs. The final section provides an overview and guidance for the use of statistical software that calculates sample sizes for clinical trials.

KEY INGREDIENTS FOR SETTING SAMPLE SIZE

Significance and Power
Suppose we are comparing two treatments: a new, experimental treatment (E) and a standard (or control) treatment (S).

FACTORS IN DETERMINING CLINICAL TRIAL SAMPLE SIZE

General Factors

Significance level (α)	Smaller value → larger sample size
Power ($1 - \beta$)	Larger value → larger sample size
Clinically relevant difference	Smaller value → larger sample size
Dilution	More → larger sample size
Allocation ratio	Unequal → usually larger sample size
Interim efficacy monitoring	More looks → larger sample size

Studies Comparing Two Means

Standard deviation in each group	Larger value → larger sample size

Studies Comparing Two Proportions

Values of the two proportions	Closer to 0.5 → larger sample size

Studies Comparing Time to Event

Accrual rate	Slower → larger sample size
Follow-up time	Shorter → larger sample size

The null hypothesis states that E and S have the same effect (there is no difference between the two). It is usually denoted by H_0.

The alternative hypothesis states that E and S have different effects (one is worse and one is better). It is usually denoted by H_A or H_1.

In general, we want to be conservative and only choose the alternative hypothesis if we are pretty sure there *is* an effect. We would rather conclude the null hypothesis is correct if there is considerable doubt. So, we specify two probabilities that reflect our levels of certainty for each decision.

- *Type I error probability* (significance level or α). This is the probability of rejecting H_0 when it is true—something we would rather not happen. So this probability is kept small: $\alpha \leq 0.05$ is the accepted upper bound.
- *Type II error probability* (β). This is the probability of not rejecting the null hypothesis when the alternative hypothesis is true. We are willing to tolerate higher probabilities for this error: $\beta \leq 0.20$. *Power* is $1 - \beta$ and should therefore always be set at 0.80 or higher.

> A good compromise position is:
> - Significance: α (two-sided) = 0.05.
> - Power: 1 − β = 0.85.

Figure 4.1 shows how α and β affect the sample size.

The alternative hypothesis may be one-sided—that is, we might only be interested in E being better than S—but this is risky, especially in superiority trials. When the Cardiac Arrhythmia Suppression Trial (CAST) was designed, investigators were sure that drugs that suppress arrhythmias could only improve survival. However, it turned out that these drugs *increased* cardiovascular mortality, and two of the three antiarrhythmic drugs were discontinued.[1,2] In light of such cautionary tales, one-sided alternative hypotheses should have a Type I error probability

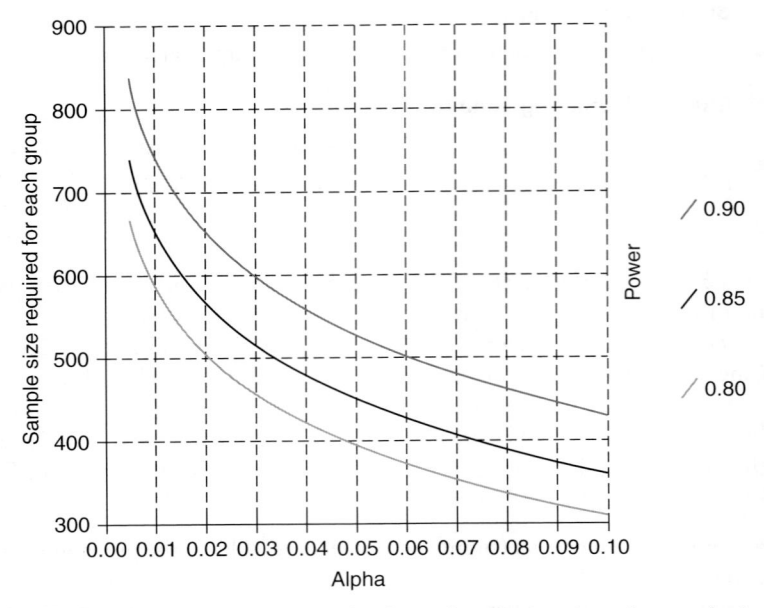

FIGURE 4.1 Effect of significance level α and power 1 − β on the sample size required for each group, when the outcome is continuous and normally distributed. Assumes a two-sided comparison trial to detect a one-point difference between group means, a five-point standard deviation within each group, and equal allocation between treatment groups.

of 0.025 (half of the two-sided Type I error). This strategy conservatively maintains the $\alpha \leq 0.05$ boundary and reduces the incentive to plan to a one-sided test. *Note:* a one-sided test with $\alpha = 0.05$ substantially reduces the total sample size—tempting, but risky.

Types of Outcomes/Endpoints That Measure Effect

The primary variable that measures the effect or difference of interest in a clinical trial is called the primary *outcome* or the primary *endpoint*. Here, we define several types of endpoints and illustrate them.

One type of endpoint is a *continuous* measure, which can take on values in a certain range. Laboratory measures, such as total cholesterol, high-density lipoprotein (HDL) cholesterol, or direct measures of low-density lipoprotein (LDL) cholesterol, are examples. Suppose we are testing a new LDL-lowering drug. Then we would randomize patients to this new drug (E) versus another LDL-lowering drug that is established as therapy (S) and treat each patient for a certain time. We would measure the participants' LDL at baseline (T_0) and at the end of the treatment period (T_1).

The simplest measure is the difference in average LDL between the two groups at the end of the trial.

However, continuous variables can be measured more than once. To adjust for baseline values, measuring at least twice will greatly increase the efficiency of the comparison, reducing the variance and thus the sample size. This can happen in two ways: either we can consider the net difference, using the difference between final and baseline LDL levels, or by adjusting the final difference for the baseline difference, using regression coefficients. In general, this last measure is the most efficient, provided the regression slope of the difference in both treatment groups is the same.[3]

A second type of outcome is *a dichotomous, yes-or-no* outcome. Death within 5 years is an example of a dichotomous endpoint with the proportion of deaths (annually) usually termed a death rate. Because this measure is an average of yes's and no's, it can be considered a simple sort of mean—a proportion. Although certain outcomes are naturally dichotomous, continuous measures are not, and when the primary outcome of a trial is really a continuous endpoint, it should be treated as such to use all the available information efficiently and keep sample size lower.

Rather than waiting to count events such as death, we could use the information more efficiently by measuring *the time to each event*—say the time to death. This becomes a *continuous* measure with the associated efficiencies. One drawback is that, for a fixed trial duration, the event will not be observed in all the subjects—many may be alive at the trial's conclusion. These are *censored* observations. In our example of death in 5 years, for subjects who are alive at the end of the trial, all we know is that their time to death is greater than the amount of time (5 years) we have followed them in the trial. Special statistical methodology has been developed for this type of truncated or censored data.[4,5] Most large cardiovascular clinical trials include censored primary endpoints, such as time to cardiovascular death. A particular subject may have died from another cause, which would be considered a *competing risk*. Those who died from another cause could be censored at their time of death. They certainly could not be observed for the cardiovascular death in which we are interested. Censoring deaths from other causes can thus introduce biased comparisons and is not technically correct. The literature on censored endpoints has been extended to consider competing risks.[6,7]

Increasingly frequently, we are interested in a number of adverse events comprising a *composite endpoint* and use the time to the first of these as the primary endpoint. In the Action to Control Cardiovascular Risk in Diabetics (ACCORD), 10,251 patients were randomly assigned to either intensive or conventional glycemia control.[8] The time to the first cardiovascular death, nonfatal myocardial infarction (MI), or nonfatal stroke is the primary endpoint. We could say that the primary outcome in the ACCORD glycemia control trial is a composite of cardiovascular death, nonfatal MI, and nonfatal stroke. Notice also that deaths from other causes are a competing risk in ACCORD.

A more complex composite endpoint was used in the Valsartan Heart Failure Trial (ValHeFT).[9] This double-blind trial randomly assigned patients to Valsartan or placebo and had two primary endpoints. These were time to death and a composite endpoint that was the time to the first of several events: death from any cause, time to hospitalization for heart failure, time to cardiac arrest with resuscitation, and time to receipt of intravenous therapy for at least 4 hours with inotropic drugs or vasodilators. In ValHeFT, there was no difference in overall survival, but the new drug showed improvement over placebo with respect to the composite endpoint.

ValHeFT also illustrates that more than one endpoint can be considered primary in a clinical trial. The simplest way to adjust the significance level for such *multiple endpoints* is to divide the overall significance level by the number of endpoints. This is known as the Bonferroni correction. It is rather conservative because it does not consider that the multiple endpoints may have some dependency. On the other hand, it is very simple

> **TYPES OF OUTCOMES IN CLINICAL TRIALS**
> - A continuous outcome can take any value between certain limits. An example is a laboratory test, which has a lower detectable limit and some upper limit.
> - A dichotomous outcome is a yes-no outcome. An example is whether or not symptoms are relieved in 24 hours. We usually compare the proportion with "yes" responses in the two groups.
> - A time-to-event outcome is continuous using all the information associated with a dichotomous event.
> - A censored outcome is continuous, but has not happened in every participant by the end of a trial. An example is time to death, when the trial ends with some people alive.
> - A composite endpoint or outcome comprises at least one of several different outcomes that are usually time-to-event (or censored). An example is time to death or to nonfatal myocardial infarction.

and does not require a complicated formula for adjustment. A more complex adjustment used in ValHeFT is the Dunn-Sîdák correction.[10]

The Trickiest Ingredient: Figuring Effect Size

How large an effect or difference should the trial be able to detect? This difference, usually expressed as a proportion of the control event rate or as a proportion of the measurement standard deviation—"a signal-to-noise ratio"—is called the *effect size*. The effect size we are interested in should be clinically relevant. It should *not* be determined statistically for a "convenient" sample size. If there have been previous studies in a similar population, one has some idea of what can be expected. However, if the previous studies have been observational (as compared to clinical trials), we might get an overly optimistic estimate.

This reduction in event rates in clinical trials, compared to observational studies, is not a well-recognized phenomenon and results from a combination of: exclusion criteria (which frequently result in eliminating sicker patients); better care from closer observation during the trial (even in the control group); and perhaps the self-selection of patients who respond well (it is well documented that about one-third of subjects will respond positively to a placebo or dummy treatment). In the SHOCK trial,[11] the sample size was conservatively set assuming a control group death rate in 30 days from cardiogenic shock complicating an acute MI of 50% and 75%, assuming the actual rate would be in that interval. At the time of planning the trial, this range seemed extremely low given a reported range of 75% to 80% in the observational series reported in the literature. The actual control group rate in the final analysis was 56%.[12]

Although considering lower effect sizes will increase sample size, this is a case of being safe rather than sorry. Remember, for fixed power and significance, the smaller the effect size to be detected, the larger the sample will have to be.

Treatment Group Strategies

Treatment group strategies are discussed in detail in Chapter 2. Several key points that directly affect sample size are noted here.

- *Control group selection* may be constrained by the comparison planned and availability of approved therapies. However, to reduce sample size, we would like clinically meaningful controls that, all other things being equal, maximize the difference to be detected. We should be sure the control and treated groups satisfy the same eligibility criteria, so that a difference between the groups can be attributed to the different treatments.
- Again, to maximize the effect size (and reduce sample size), we would like to choose the most effective version of the *experimental therapy*. We may specify that the dose of the new treatment is to be determined by individual characteristics. However, if we randomize to more than two groups, we are likely to need a larger sample size than if we have a two-group design.

Subject Accrual

A critical part of undertaking a clinical trial is recruiting an adequate number of subjects. Trialists are often optimistic about the proportion of their patients who will enroll in the trial among those who are eligible, and often they underestimate the difficulty of accruing patients in the time frame that has been planned. Because trial duration depends on the time it will take to accrue the required number of subjects, it is important to have good estimates of the number that each site can accrue in a given time period. It may be worthwhile to have sites submit the numbers of subjects in the previous year or two who would have been eligible for a trial that is now being planned. A cautious trialist would estimate that no more than 50% (sometimes many fewer) of those eligible will actually enroll. It is also advisable to have more sites to accrue subjects than appears to be needed. At the worst, accrual will take less time than anticipated and the trial will end earlier than expected.

Because it is a frequent experience that accrual takes more time than anticipated, it is wise to consider the implications of this when the trial is designed, not when the 3 years of anticipated accrual have yielded half the number of patients expected! One should monitor actual versus expected accrual overall and by site so that problems can be identified (and solved) early on. Chapter 9 discusses this issue as well as how to maximize follow-up.

Trial Duration

In a clinical trial with time-to-an-event as the endpoint, there will be more events (and therefore more power) if trial subjects are followed longer on average. The trialist should also consider if the trial is long enough for sufficient events to happen. Certainly, assumptions about accrual duration and follow-up duration should be varied to assess their influence on sample size.

Some "event" trials are designed to continue to follow patients until a certain prespecified number of events occur, and if events occur quickly, as in certain cancer trials, perhaps the target sample size could be decreased. In other trials where most events will occur after accrual is completed and estimates of event rates are uncertain, rather than a fixed duration trial, one could continue the trial until a certain number of events occurs. If the funding is flexible enough to accommodate the certain cost of varying trial duration, this type of trial design will retain its power.

Dilution (Including Crossovers)

If not included up front as a key ingredient, dilution can result in an entirely inadequate sample size because of its impact on **effect size**. It is better to be very conservative and have the luxury of increased power than to have to terminate the trial for unattainable sample size and, therefore, power.

Dilution of the effect size occurs when subjects, for whatever reason, do not complete the treatment according to protocol. Typical situations for dilution are:

- Subjects, or their physicians, may refuse the therapy to which they were randomly assigned, choosing another therapy offered in the trial, something else, or nothing at all.
- Subjects may stop the assigned therapy early or vary the dose (particularly if burdensome or with uncomfortable side effects).

- For an escalating dose, median dose achieved may be much lower than initially projected, thus diminishing the effect size.
- Slow initial accrual, resulting in a lower median follow-up, will result in a smaller effect size, unless accommodated in the initial calculations.
- A substantial proportion of ineligible subjects (> 5%) may be randomized, potentially diluting the "intent-to-treat" analysis when they do not complete treatment; and/or are unsuitable for demonstrating a treatment effect (e.g., too sick, too healthy, do not actually have the condition being studied).
- Loss to follow-up may be substantial (see Chapter 9).

These six reasons—and variants of them—can result in reduced effect sizes and thus inadequate power, if not included, conservatively, in the original sample size calculation.

The first reason, when subjects end up on a trial therapy to which they were not assigned, is usually termed *crossovers*. This form of dilution can be particularly damaging if not included generously in the sample size calculation. An excellent example is provided by the Magnesium in Coronaries trial (MAGIC).[13] In designing this large, simple trial, an 11% dilution effect (including both crossovers and ineligibles) was assumed in each treatment arm given little available prior information. The actual dilution was less than 1%. Because the trial was designed with 10,400 subjects to have 90% power to detect a 20% relative treatment effect in 30-day mortality and the crossover rate was so low, the Data and Safety Monitoring Board (DSMB) recommended decreasing the sample size of the trial to 6,100 based on blinded data after approximately one-third accrual. Power remained at 90%. While the crossovers were considerably overestimated, it was clearly better to be safe, especially given that the trial was subsequently expanded internationally after initiation in North America only.

Crossovers occur in both experimental and control treatment groups, particularly when the therapies are available outside the trial. This is an increasing problem with trials of devices or procedures. Patients may crossover to the standard therapy if randomized to the experimental, and vice versa.

Dilution can occur at different times in different treatment groups. When a surgical procedure is compared to a pharmaceutical therapy, crossovers or dropouts from the surgery occur early, while later crossovers will occur on drug therapy. In general, assuming that dilution occurs early provides larger sample sizes that can be retained for greater power.

HOW CROSSOVERS DILUTE THE EFFECT SIZE FOR TWO TREATMENT GROUPS: EXPERIMENTAL (E) AND STANDARD (S)

	E	S	Effect Size
Hypothesized outcome rates	50%	30%	20%

Crossover Scenario I

5% ⟶

Outcome rates: 0.95 (50) + 0.05 (30)
= 49%   30%   19%

Crossover Scenario II

5% ⟶

⟵ 10%

Outcome rates: 0.95 (50) + 0.05 (30)   0.9 (30) + 0.1 (50)
= 49%   = 32%   17%

It is strongly recommended that researchers investigate the impact on effect size (and thus on sample size) of varying the assumptions on sources of dilution—a sensitivity analysis of dilution assumptions.

SAMPLE SIZE FOR SUPERIORITY TRIALS: SIMPLEST CASES

Several classic papers describe sample size calculations for two-arm randomized controlled trials.[14–20] In this section we will deal with equal sample sizes per treatment group for three problems: the difference in means (with unknown but equal variances), the difference in proportions, and the hazard ratio for survival distributions. We restrict our discussion to two-sided tests ($\alpha = 0.05$).

Sample Size for the Difference in Means

The simplest case for setting sample size involves the difference in means, with known and equal variance (σ^2) in each group.

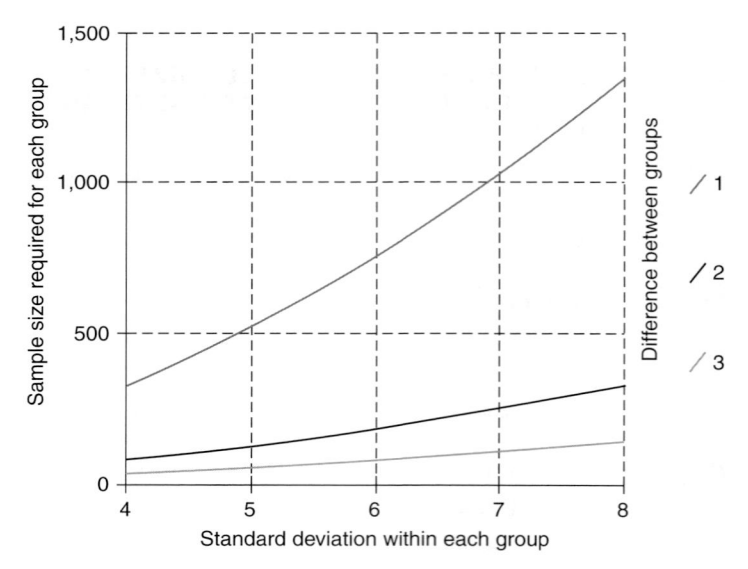

FIGURE 4.2 Effect of the standard deviation within each group and the treatment group difference on the sample size required for each group, for a continuous, normally distributed outcome. Assumes a two-sided comparison trial with 90% power, α = 0.05, and equal allocation between the two groups.

When σ^2 is unknown (and equal in the two treatment groups), we can set sample size by estimating σ^2. Cohen[21] provides extensive sample size tables for an effect size parameter δ/σ, which he calls the *standardized difference* (also known as a *signal-to-noise ratio*). A more complex but improved approach is provided by Guenther.[22]

Example

The African-American Heart Failure Trial (A-HeFT) used a composite of death from any cause, hospitalization, and change in quality of life as its primary endpoint.[23] The components of the composite endpoint were scored so that everyone received values between −3 and +2. For the sample size calculation, data from a previous trial, V-HeFT, were used. The study was designed to have a power of 0.80 to detect a difference between groups equivalent to 0.228 of a standard deviation when hypothesis testing was undertaken at the α = 0.05 level. The authors note that the anticipated standard deviation of the composite score, again based on their previous trial, was between 0.5 and 1, so that 0.228

standard deviation was less than one-quarter of a unit of their score function. The sample size per treatment arm (n) = 302 subjects. The A-HeFT trial was designed with 300 subjects per arm.

It is worth noting that the composite endpoint in A-HeFT was defined so that everyone had the value 0 at baseline. This avoided having to consider reasonable estimates for the (common) standard deviation of the changes from baseline for the outcome measure in the two treatment groups.

For a trial comparing two means, the effect size is the ratio of the treatment difference to the standard deviation. Figure 4.2 shows the effect of the standard deviation and treatment difference on the sample size.

Sample Size for the Difference in Proportions

Suppose that the trial outcome can be expressed as the proportion of patients in each treatment group who have a certain characteristic at the end of the trial. Examples are the proportion of responses to treatment (e.g., a new cancer chemotherapy regimen versus conventional chemotherapy for a solid tumor, such as small-cell lung cancer) in a fixed time period, say 4 months; or the proportion of patients who are disease free at 3 years.

Casagrande et al.[14] provide a formula for the sample size in each of two treatment groups.

The sample size depends not only on the difference between the proportions, or the ratio of the proportions, but also on the proportion in the control group. For example, a study to detect a difference between proportions of 0.2 and 0.3 will need fewer subjects than a study to detect a difference between proportions of 0.45 and 0.55.

Figure 4.3 shows the effect on sample size of the control proportion and the difference between proportions. Figure 4.4 shows the effect of the control proportion and the ratio between proportions.

Setting Sample Size for the Hazard Ratio

The most commonplace example of censored data is survival data, although time to any event will use the same statistical approach. When the time to death is compared between two groups, the assumption of *proportional hazards* is usually made. The hazard function at time t is the instantaneous probability of death at time t. The proportional hazards assumption says that the ratio of the hazard function for each subject (λ), whether he or she is given the new treatment (E) or the control treatment (S), is a constant. *For survival data, power is a function of the number of deaths, not the number of subjects.*

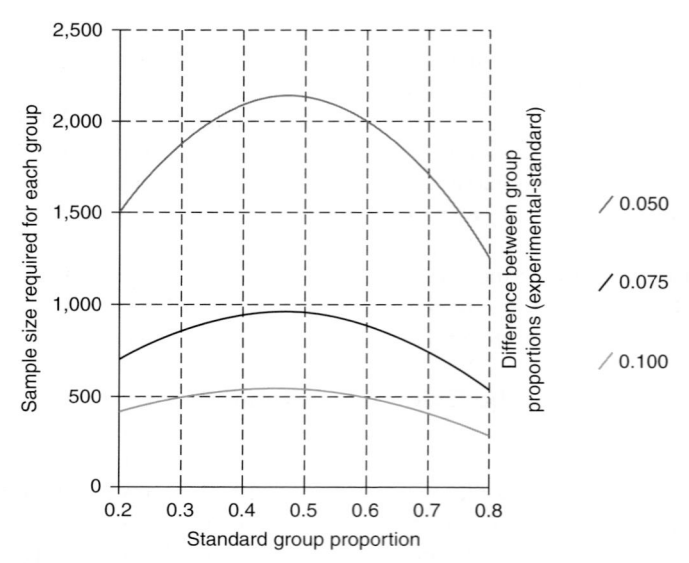

FIGURE 4.3 Effect of control group proportion, and difference between proportions, on the sample size required for each group. Assumes a two-sided comparison trial using a chi-squared test, with equal allocation between the groups, 90% power, and $\alpha = 0.05$.

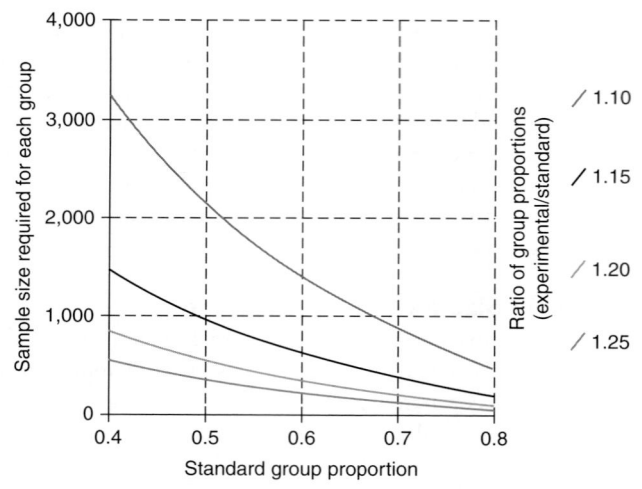

FIGURE 4.4 Effect of control group proportion, and ratio of proportions, on the sample size required for each group. Assumes a two-sided comparison trial using chi-squared test, with equal allocation between the groups, 90% power, and $\alpha = 0.05$.

Let the proportion of deaths in the control group (S) be p_S and suppose we are interested in detecting a *percentage reduction of r* in the new treatment group (E). *Sometimes r is called the effect size.* Thus p_E, the proportion of deaths in E, would be $p_S(1-r)$. Under the proportional hazards assumption, there is a relationship between λ, the hazard ratio we wish to detect, and p_S and r. Thus comparisons of survival distributions may be expressed in terms of p_S and either r or λ.

Freedman[19] provides tables of the number of patients required in clinical trials with a survival endpoint using the logrank test, expressed in terms of the proportions alive at the end of the trial. Freedman recommends guessing the proportion of patients event-free at the minimum follow-up time in the less favorable group, and setting sample size based on the resulting minimum difference considered clinically worthwhile to detect. He shows how to approximate the total number of events required. His tables give both the total number of subjects needed, and the total number of events for these conservative assumptions. For entries not included in the tables, Freedman[19] gives an approximate formula.

Note that for a fixed number of subjects, the longer the follow-up period, the greater number of deaths (events) that will occur. Also, if the number of subjects is accrued rapidly and the follow-up period is fixed, each will be followed up for a longer period of time, and so a greater number of deaths will occur.

Example

The Prevention of Events with Angiotensin-Converting Enzyme inhibition (PEACE) trial[24] compared an angiotensin-converting-enzyme (ACE) inhibitor, trandilopril, to placebo in patients with stable coronary heart disease and with slightly reduced or normal left ventricular function. Both treatment groups also received modern conventional therapy, which included cholesterol and blood pressure lowering medications as appropriate. The primary question was whether adding an ACE inhibitor in those with early heart disease would decrease the likelihood of a composite endpoint of cardiovascular death, nonfatal myocardial infarction, and coronary revascularization. Even with a proposed median follow-up time of 4.8 years, relatively few in the control group (19%) were anticipated to have these events. Trandilopril would be considered effective in this population if the percent with events was reduced by 18%, that is, to $0.19(1-0.18) = 0.1558$. For setting sample size, methods for censored data were appropriate. For $\alpha = 0.05$ and 90% power, we would need about 888 total events, or a total sample of over 5,000. The illustration is approximate, in that it does not consider the time it takes to accrue this number of patients or the impact of various dilution factors.

PEACE further assumed a drop in to treatment of 15% (because other ACE inhibitors are available by prescription) and a drop out from treatment of 15% (because these patients are not very ill and because ACE inhibitors have side effects). This increased the sample size to 8,100 patients, using the method of Shih[25] (discussed in the last section of this chapter), which allows more precise assumptions to be made, including duration and pattern of accrual and follow-up, as well as patterns of drop in and drop out. The actual sample-size calculation assumed a 15% rate of discontinuation of active treatment and a 15% rate of crossover to active treatment occurring uniformly over the trial duration.[24]

SETTING SAMPLE SIZE FOR EQUIVALENCE AND NONINFERIORITY TRIAL DESIGNS

We use the results above for superiority trials to discuss sample size calculations for equivalence or noninferiority trials, where rather than demonstrating that one treatment is superior to another, the goal is to show that the two treatment groups differ by less than some small amount (Δ), or that the new treatment (E) is no worse than the standard (S) (see Chapter 2 for an expanded discussion of these trials).[26–28]

The statistical analysis and sample size calculation for noninferiority and equivalence trials are usually based on the confidence interval (CI) approach. The required sample size for a noninferiority trial depends on the prespecified error rates (α, β) and margin of equivalence or noninferiority Δ.[26,29] This margin Δ is often chosen as the largest value that would be clinically acceptable and it should be smaller than a clinically important effect chosen to test superiority of a treatment against placebo. Thus, an equivalence trial usually requires a considerably larger sample size than a superiority trial.

In noninferiority trials, dilution can make two treatments more similar, and hence investigators must pay special attention to trial conduct and analysis. The *on-treatment* and *per-protocol* analysis might be more desirable as the primary analysis than the intention-to-treat (ITT) analysis. However, some argue to use the ITT analysis for the primary analysis to protect against possible unknown biases from *on-treatment* analysis. Some studies plan up front to check for superiority if noninferiority is demonstrated. Using ITT can facilitate this comparison. See Garrett[30] for an extensive discussion on analysis of equivalence trials.

Example

The Rosiglitazone Evaluated for Cardiac Outcomes and Regulation of Glycaemia in Diabetes (RECORD) trial is an active controlled, noninferiority trial in type 2 diabetic patients with inadequate blood glucose control.[31] This randomized study was designed to compare the add-on rosiglitazone group (E) with the standard therapy group (S), which received a combination of metformin plus sulfonylurea. RECORD used hospitalization or death from cardiovascular causes as its primary endpoint. The rosiglitazone group (E) was designated as noninferior to S if the upper limit of the two-sided 95% CI of the hazard ratio for the primary endpoint was below 1.20 on completion of the study. An event rate of 11% per year was assumed for S. Thus the overall event rate of 0.503 for S and the absolute maximum event rate difference $\Delta = 0.0649$ can be estimated for the trial, assuming a median of 6 years follow-up. The total sample required for 99% power would be approximately 3,750. RECORD was actually designed with a total of 4,000 patients after taking account of likely loss to follow-up.

SAMPLE SIZE FOR OTHER COMPLEX TRIAL DESIGNS

Here we consider cluster randomized trials, where the unit of randomization is a group, rather than an individual; repeated measures designs, where a certain variable is measured at several time points in each treatment group and the goal is to use all of the information to determine if the two treatment effects differ; and crossover trials, where unlike in the parallel group design, each subject is randomized to receive a sequence of treatments at different fixed-length time periods during the course of the trial, thus serving as his or her own control.

Cluster Unit Trials

For certain prevention trials, it may be more convenient or logistically make more sense to implement the interventions in preexisting groupings (e.g., in communities, clinics, or worksites) rather than in individuals. In dietary or lifestyle intervention studies, the use of a cluster (such as school or family) as the unit of randomization may minimize the risk of contamination, compared to trials in which individuals within the same cluster may be randomized to different interventions. Examples of cluster randomization trials include school-based intervention trials, such as the Child and Adolescent Trial for Cardiovascular Health (CATCH),[32] and community-based intervention trials, such as the Rapid Early Action for Coronary Treatment (REACT) trial.[33]

Cluster trials pose a number of problems in the design and sample size calculation. Because the unit of randomization is a cluster, to have desirable power for the statistical analysis, *a cluster randomized trial must include an adequate number of clusters*. Then the total number of subjects available equals the number of clusters multiplied by the average cluster size. Outcome measurements in each cluster are made directly at the cluster level or are aggregated data from individuals in the cluster.

The power of the trial depends more on the number of clusters than on the number of subjects per cluster. Increasing the cluster *size* may not have substantial impact on the power, especially for clusters with large intracluster correlations between individuals (ρ). Donner and Klar[34] provided a useful rule of thumb that, for fixed numbers of clusters, the gains in power will be rather modest once the number of subjects per cluster exceeds $1/\rho$. Hence, to reduce the effort and cost of data collection, subjects may be randomly subsampled within the large clusters. Values of ρ have been reported for a variety of populations and outcomes.[35,36]

A key issue in the design of a cluster randomized trial is how to measure the cluster outcomes. Cohort design and cross-sectional design for the per-cluster measures are two main approaches. In the cohort approach, a cohort of individuals (or all individuals) within each cluster is followed and measured over time during the trial. In the cross-sectional approach, samples are selected independently within each cluster at each measurement time point. Feldman and McKinlay (1994)[37] unify these two approaches in a single mixed-effects model and provide excellent examples of the needed parameter values from recent trials. McKinlay[38]

KEY ISSUES IN DETERMINING THE SAMPLE SIZE FOR CLUSTER RANDOMIZED TRIALS

- The number of clusters is the *operating* sample size for power calculations
- The level at which outcomes are measured is a key factor
- Method of measuring cluster outcomes: Cohort vs. Cross-sectional design

extends this unified model to the calculation of sample sizes for cluster unit trials. The choice of cohort versus cross-sectional sampling with clusters depends on the length of follow-up and the rates of migration in and out of the clusters (dilution effect).[37]

For some trials, the number of clusters may be limited. To minimize imbalance and ensure comparability across the intervention groups, stratified and matched-pair designs may be adopted based on the characteristics of clusters. Some large cluster randomized trials may also contain multiple levels of units, including the primary randomized clusters (e.g., communities or schools) and lower-lever units (e.g., neighborhoods or classroom). Then intracluster correlations at different levels need to be considered. Further details on the design and methodologic issues of complex cluster randomization trials can be found in textbooks[32,35,36] and in recent review papers.[34,39]

Example

The Child and Adolescent Trial for Cardiovascular Health (CATCH) was a clustered randomized trial with school-based educational and environmental interventions in elementary school children.[32] The intervention was aimed at promoting heart-healthy habits such as low fat and salt consumption and physical exercise. The trial primary endpoint was the serum total cholesterol change in children, because it would be free of reporting bias. CATCH used a cohort design, in which the study cohort was defined to be those students who underwent a baseline cholesterol measurement. Those students migrating out of CATCH schools were tracked in order to obtain their cholesterol measurements at the end of the study. In the CATCH sample size calculation,[32] intracluster correlations were estimated based on a prior observational study in one of the study centers. The calculation yielded an inflation factor of 1.50 and a total of 96 schools to detect a 5.1 mg/dL difference in cholesterol between the intervention and control groups with nearly 90% power.

Repeated Measures Designs

In *repeated measures studies* or *longitudinal studies,* investigators may be primarily interested in comparing different treatment groups in terms of their rates of change (slope) or their mean responses over time. Repeated measures of response may include blood pressure, laboratory measurements, lung function, and quality-of-life scores. Because repeated observations for the same subject are usually positively correlated, it has been shown that repeated measures designs are potentially more efficient and powerful, compared to designs that only use the measurement at the final visit or the change in the measures from baseline to the final visit. However, the design and analysis of repeated measures studies are more complex. Investigators need to determine not only the number of subjects to enroll in the study but also the study duration and the number and spacing of repeated measurements per subject. In general, responses are assumed to be linear over time.[40]

Example

Consider a trial to test two treatments to lower the LDL cholesterol level. Four visits are planned at 0, 0.5, 1, and 2 years since the trial inception. Assume also that the study is planned for 85% power, two-sided significance 0.05, a treatment difference of 5 mg/dL per year, a within-subject inter-observation correlation ρ of 0.5, and the standard deviation of LDL levels of 25 mg/dL. Using these parameters, the total sample size would be 206. If we assume a larger ρ of 0.75, then the total sample size would reduce by half to 104. Thus it would be conservative (and wise) not to assume an extremely high correlation in the sample size calculation.

Rather than comparing the rate of change (slope) of a continuous response, suppose that investigators are interested in comparing the mean responses or the mean response rates over all follow-up visits for the two treatment groups. Then the calculation for the number of subjects would be similar to the calculation for the number of clusters in cluster randomized trials, as a single individual may be considered as a cluster unit with correlated measurements.

Other methods of sample size calculations for repeated measures have been proposed, corresponding to different analytic models such as the two-stage mixed model analysis[41–43] and the generalized estimating equations approaches.[44,45]

Crossover Trials

Crossover trials are particularly useful to assess the within-patient treatment difference by giving each subject all treatments under comparison at different periods of time during a trial. This design is frequently used to compare patient preference for different short-acting treatments in studies of certain chronic diseases such as asthma and hypertension.

Because each subject serves as his or her own control in a crossover trial, the variability of the treatment differences is reduced, and it might

ADVANTAGES AND DISADVANTAGES OF CROSSOVER TRIALS
- Advantages: reduced sample size and improved subject recruitment
- Disadvantages: residual or carry-over effects of treatments and subject dropouts

require a much smaller sample size compared to a parallel group design. It may improve recruitment over parallel placebo-controlled trials, as each subject will have a chance to receive the active or novel treatment at a certain period during the trial. However, factors such as the carry-over effect and subject dropout increase the complexity in trial design and analysis. Because it is difficult to estimate carry-over effects, it is recommended to use crossover trials for treatments with negligible carry-over effects or to allow enough time between treatment periods to *wash out* the effect of the previous treatment.

The simplest crossover trial uses the two-treatment two-period (two-by-two) design, or the AB/BA design. In a two-by-two crossover trial, one group of n patients receives treatment A followed by treatment B (sometimes, after a washout period), and the other group receives the treatments in the reverse order. Assume the null hypothesis is no difference between the treatments A and B, against the alternative that A and B differ. For crossover trials with a continuous outcome, the difference in average outcomes under the two treatments is commonly used, for which the simple paired t-test can be applied.

The design and sample size calculation for more complex crossover trials with three or more treatments can be found in Jones and Kenwood[46] and Senn.[47]

Example
The Dietary Approaches to Stop Hypertension (DASH)-Sodium trial was a randomized crossover trial to study the effect of different levels of dietary sodium on blood pressure.[48] Participants with higher than optimal blood pressure or stage 1 hypertension were assigned to a certain dietary pattern at each of three sodium levels (higher, intermediate, lower) for 30 days. The primary outcome was systolic blood pressure (SBP) measured at the end of each intervention feeding period. In the run-in feeding period, participants were fed at the higher sodium level because this level is the typical level of U.S. consumption. The run-in

period was designed to identify and exclude those persons unlikely to adhere to the dietary requirements and to establish the energy level needed to maintain weight. Participants then entered the three 30-day controlled sodium intake feeding periods in a random order. The three feeding periods could be separated by up to 5 days as the carryover effects from one feeding to the next were expected to be minimal for the outcomes.

Suppose that the standard deviation (SD) of SBP differences is estimated to be 10 mm Hg; then the total sample size would be 100 to have 85% power to detect a difference of 3 mm Hg in SBP between the high and low sodium levels. To illustrate the savings in the sample size with a crossover trial, we can also consider a parallel group design for the same treatment effect. If we can assume the SD for SBP change from baseline for each group to be the same (10 mm Hg), then the total sample size would be 400—four times the size required for the crossover trial. Note that if the study is powered to compare all three sodium levels, we also need to adjust for multiple testing in the sample size calculation.

SOFTWARE

A number of commercial software packages are available for sample size and power calculations such as nQuery Advisor by Statistical solutions (http://www.statsol.ie) and PASS by NCSS (http://www.ncss.com/pass.html). These software tools can compute the sample sizes for different types of tests and endpoints with user choices of allowable error rates (Type I error and power) and treatment effect size. In addition, other conditions such as loss to follow-up, other dilution factors, and staggered entry during a period of accrual can also be specified. Two new procedures in the Statistical Analysis System (SAS),[49] the POWER and GLMPOWER procedures, can perform the analysis for a variety of statistical tests. Statistical analysis packages such as SAS, S-PLUS, and R can also be easily programmed to determine the sample size and power.

Certain freeware is available for sample size calculations (see Piantadosi[50] for a review). We have used the programs provided by Hsieh[51] and Piantadosi (http://www.cancerbiostats.onc.jhmi.edu/software.cfm). An elegant SAS macro program that considers accrual patterns, drop in, drop out, loss to follow-up in a time-dependent fashion was written by Shih.[25] This program refines earlier work by allowing very complex assumptions to be made in estimating sample size. One should keep in mind that the more assumptions that are made, the more likely it is that

> **FEATURES TO LOOK FOR IN SAMPLE SIZE SOFTWARE:**
> - Which study designs does the software handle?
> - Do the results agree with results from published formulas?
> - How easy is it to use the software?
> - Does it format the results in a way that is easy to interpret (table formats, graphs, etc)?
> - Does it have good documentation or help files?
> - Does it have good user support?
> - How expensive is it?

some of them will turn out to be incorrect! In general, "freeware" comes with less documentation than commercial software and is more likely to contain some errors that a naive user would not notice.

With the help of computer programs and software, sensitivity analysis and statistical simulation can be easily performed to study the impact on the sample size and power when investigators vary the design parameters and trial assumptions. A consultation with a statistician is also recommended.

REFERENCES

1. Bigger JT Jr. The events surrounding the removal of encainide and flecainide from the Cardiac Arrhythmia Suppression Trial (CAST) and why CAST is continuing with moricizine. *J Am Coll Cardiol.* 1990;15:243–245.
2. Friedman LM, Bristow JD, Hallstrom A, et al. Data monitoring in the cardiac arrhythmia suppression trial. *Online J Curr Clin Trials.* 1993; doc no. 79.
3. Snedecor GW, Cochran WG. *Statistical Methods.* Iowa State University Press; 8th edition Ames: Iowa, 1989.
4. Miller RG. *Survival Analysis.* New York: Wiley-Interscience; 1998.
5. Lee ET, Wang JW. *Statistical Methods for Survival Data Analysis.* 3rd ed. New York: Wiley-Interscience; 2003.
6. Gray RJ. A class of K-sample tests for comparing the cumulative incidence of a competing risk. *Ann Stat.* 1988;16:1141–1154.
7. Gooley TA, Leisenring W, Crowley J, et al. Estimation of failure probabilities in the presence of competing risks: new representations of old estimators. *Stat Med.* 1999;18:695–706.
8. The ACCORD Study Group. Action to Control Cardiovascular Risk in Diabetes (ACCORD) Trial: design and methods. *Am J Cardiol.* 2007; 99:21i–33i.

9. Cohn JN, Tognoni G. A randomized trial of the angiotensin-receptor blocker valsartan in chronic heart failure. *N Engl J Med.* 2001;345:1667–1675.
10. Hochberg Y, Tamhane AC. *Multiple Comparison Procedures.* New York: Wiley-Interscience; 1987.
11. Hochman JS, Sleeper LA, Godfrey E, et al. Should we emergently revascularize occluded coronaries for cardiogenic shock: an international randomized trial of emergency PTCA/CABG: trial design. *Am Heart J.* 1999;137:313–321.
12. Hochman JS, Sleeper LA, Webb JG, et al. Early revascularization in acute myocardial infarction complicated by cardiogenic shock. *N Engl J Med.* 1999;341:625–634.
13. The Magnesium in Coronaries (MAGIC) trial investigators. Early administration of intravenous magnesium to high-risk patients with acute myocardial infarction in the Magnesium in Coronaries (MAGIC) trial: a randomized controlled trial. *Lancet.* 2002:360:1189–1196.
14. Casagrande JT, Pike MC, Smith PG. An improved approximate formula for calculating sample sizes for comparing two binomial distributions. *Biometrics.* 1978;34:483–486.
15. Fleiss J, Tytun A, Ury S. A simple approximation for calculating sample sizes for comparing independent proportions. *Biometrics.* 1980;36:343–346.
16. Fleiss JL, Levin B, Paik MC. *Statistical Methods for Rates and Proportions.* 3rd ed. New York: Wiley-Interscience; 2003.
17. Lachin JM. Introduction to sample size determination and power analysis for clinical trials. *Control Clin Trials.* 1981;2:93–113.
18. Rubinstein L, Gail M, Santner T. Planning the duration of a comparative clinical trial with loss to follow-up and a period of continued observation. *J Chron Dis.* 1981;34:469–479.
19. Freedman L. Tables of the number of patients required in clinical trials using the logrank test. *Stat Med.* 1982;1:121–129.
20. Schoenfeld DA. Sample-size formula for the proportional-hazards regression model. *Biometrics.* 1983;39:499–503.
21. Cohen J. *Statistical Power Analysis for the Behavioral Sciences.* 2nd ed. Hillsdale, NJ: Erlbaum; 1988.
22. Guenther WC. Sample size formulas for normal theory T-tests. *Am Statistician.* 1981;35:243–244.
23. Franciosa JA, Taylor AL, Cohn JN, et al. African-American Heart Failure Trial (A-HeFT): rationale, design, and methodology. *J Card Fail.* 2002; 8:128–135.
24. Braunwald E, Domanski MJ, Fowler SE, et al. Angiotensin-converting-enzyme inhibition in stable coronary artery disease. *N Engl J Med.* 2004;351:2058–2068.
25. Shih J. Sample size estimation for complex clinical trials. *Control Clin Trials.* 1995;16:395–407.
26. Jones B, Jarvis P, Lewis JA, et al. Trials to assess equivalence: the importance of rigorous methods. *BMJ.* 1996;313:36–39.

27. Piaggio G, Elbourne DR, Altman DG, et al. CONSORT group. Reporting of noninferiority and equivalence randomized trials: an extension of the CONSORT statement. *JAMA*. 2006;295:1152–1160.
28. Blackwelder WC. Current issues in clinical equivalence trials. *J Dent Res*. 2004;83:C113–C115.
29. Blackwelder WC. "Proving the null Hypothesis" in clinical trials. *Control Clin Trials*. 1982;3:345–353.
30. Garrett AD. Therapeutic equivalence: fallacies and falsification. *Stat Med*. 2003;22:741–762.
31. Home PD, Pocock SJ, Beck-Nielsen H, et al. RECORD study group. Rosiglitazone evaluated for cardiovascular outcomes: an interim analysis. *N Engl J Med*. 2007;357:28–38.
32. Zucker DM. Design and analysis of cluster randomization trials. In: Geller N, ed. *Advances in Clinical Trial Biostatistics*. New York: Dekker; 2004.
33. Luepker RV, Raczynski JM, Osganian S, et al. Effect of a community intervention on patient delay and emergency medical service use in acute coronary heart disease: the Rapid Early Action for Coronary Treatment (REACT) trial. *JAMA*. 2000;284:60–67.
34. Donner A, Klar N. Pitfalls of and controversies in cluster randomization trials. *Am J Public Health*. 2004;94:416–422.
35. Murray DM. *Design and Analysis of Group Randomized Trials*. Oxford: Oxford University Press; 1998.
36. Donner A, Klar N. *Design and Analysis of Cluster Randomization Trials in Health Research*. London: Arnold; 2000.
37. Feldman HA, McKinlay SM. Cohort versus cross-sectional design in large field trials: Precision, sample size, and a unifying model. *Stat Med*. 1994;13:61–78.
38. McKinlay SM. Cost-efficient designs of cluster unit trials. *Prev Med*. 1994;23:606–611.
39. Campbell MJ, Donner A, Klar N. Developments in cluster randomized trials and statistics in medicine. *Stat Med*. 2007;26:2–19.
40. Diggle PJ, Heagerty P, Liang K-Y, et al. *Analysis of Longitudinal Data*. 2nd ed. Oxford: Oxford University Press; 2002.
41. Schlesselman JJ. Planning a longitudinal study. I. Sample size determination. *J Chron Dis*. 1973;26:553–560.
42. Schlesselman JJ. Planning a longitudinal study. II. Frequency of measurement and study duration. *J Chron Dis*. 1973;26:561–570.
43. Fitzmaurice G, Laird N, Ware J. *Applied Longitudinal Analysis*. New York: Wiley; 2004.
44. Liu G, Liang KY. Sample size calculations for studies with correlated observations. *Biometrics*. 1997;53:937–947.
45. Rochon J. Application of GEE procedures for sample size calculations in repeated measures experiments. *Stat Med*. 1998;17:1643–1658.
46. Jones B, Kenwood MG. *Design and Analysis of Cross-Over Trials*. London: Chapman & Hall/CRC; 1989.

47. Senn S. *Cross-over Trials in Clinical Research*. New York: Wiley; 1993.
48. Sacks FM, Svetkey LP, Vollmer WM, et al. Effects on blood pressure of reduced dietary sodium and the Dietary Approaches to Stop Hypertension (DASH) diet. DASH-Sodium Collaborative Research Group. *N Engl J Med*. 2001;344:3–10.
49. SAS Institute. *SAS/STAT User's Guide*, version 9.1.3. Cary, NC: SAS Institute; 2003.
50. Piantadosi S. *Clinical Trials: A Methodologic Perspective*. 2nd ed. New York: Wiley-Interscience; 2005.
51. Hsieh F. SSIZE: a sample size program for clinical and epidemiologic studies. *Am Statistician*. 1991;45:338.

FURTHER READING

Altman DG. *Practical Statistics for Medical Research*. London: Chapman & Hall; 1991.

Fleiss JL, Levin B, Paik MC. *Statistical Methods for Rates and Proportions*. 3rd ed. New York: Wiley-Interscience; 2003.

Friedman LM, Furberg CD, DeMets DL. *Fundamentals of Clinical Trials*. 3rd ed. New York: Springer; 1998.

Geller NL, ed. *Advances in Clinical Trials Biostatistics*. New York: Dekker; 2004.

Piantadosi S. *Clinical Trials: A Methodologic Perspective*. 2nd ed. New York: Wiley-Interscience; 2005.

CHAPTER 5

Analytic Approach and Methods

LYNN A. SLEEPER

This chapter discusses approaches to the analysis of data from randomized clinical trials and provides a conceptual overview of statistical methods that are appropriate for specific trial designs and types of outcome measures.

Analysis of trial data occurs at nearly all stages of a study. The first section describes the goals of and guidelines for analysis at each of these stages: data cleaning, interim analysis of trial data, and final analysis.

There are several issues related to the analysis of randomized clinical trial data that are applicable to all types of study designs and outcome measures. The next section discusses approaches for both primary and secondary analysis of results, the handling of data in interim analyses, as well as approaches for assessing the impact of missing data on inferences made from trial findings.

The specific statistical method used for analysis of trial data varies according to the type of study outcome and the trial design. The final section provides a brief overview of appropriate statistical methods according to type of outcome, effective reporting methods for trial results, and guidelines for interpretation of findings.

STAGES OF ANALYSIS

Analysis of trial data is an ongoing process, from the accrual phase to the end of all follow-up. There are three main stages: data cleaning, interim analysis of outcomes, and final analysis. It is important for trial integrity to keep in mind that:

- Early and ongoing review of data quality is important, but *should not involve analysis of treatment differences.*

- Interim analysis encompasses scrutiny of enrollment and protocol compliance, as well as prespecified reporting of outcomes.
- Outcome data analysis by treatment arm *should only be viewed by designated statisticians and an appointed monitoring board.*
- Whether the findings are reported in aggregate or by treatment arm depends on the timing and type of trial outcome.

Stage I

In stage I, as subjects are being recruited, it is important to review accruing baseline and treatment administration data for ranges of variables, variation among sites, and baseline differences by treatment arm.

Simple analysis of the distributions of baseline study measurements early on and continuing throughout the trial is important. One might learn that the range for a novel measurement is much greater than originally estimated, and data entry systems could be modified to accept a broader validation range, increasing speed of data entry by decreasing the frequency of required documentation necessary for overrides of expected ranges. In a similar vein, a measurement could be common for one population (e.g., adults), but perhaps novel for the trial population (e.g., children), and examination of its distribution in the sample provides helpful information on minimum and maximum values. Another reason for examining distributions of data is to identify potential problems with equipment (measurement error) or data entry errors related to measurement units.

Stratified data analyses are also revealing and can suggest actions needed to continue protocol implementation. Differences between sites may be expected—for example, patient populations may differ due to referral patterns. However, variation by site may also reflect differential implementation of the protocol, indicating a need for retraining or recalibration of equipment. Last, examination of baseline differences by treatment arm are acceptable and important to monitor. If such differences are observed, it should be kept in mind that as the sample size increases, random differences should dissipate and no action is usually necessary. However, if a difference is observed in a variable that is known to be strongly related to outcome, trial investigators may want to consider adding it as a stratification factor for the randomization scheme. It should be noted that *comparisons of post-baseline study outcomes by treatment group are not conducted in stage I.*

These aspects of becoming familiar with the data will greatly enhance the efficiency of trial closeout. However, study outcome measures post-baseline cannot be reported or used for treatment group comparisons in this stage.

Stage II

In stage II, interim analysis of trial data is conducted to assess trial performance with regard to:

"LOOK AND LEARN"
1. Feasibility of enrollment.
2. Compliance with the protocol.

"RESTRICTED ACCESS ONLY"
3. Estimation of overall event rates and variance of outcome measures.
4. Safety of new treatments.
5. Efficacy of treatments.

It should be noted that because assessment of data quality is an ongoing process as data accrue, stage I data cleaning activities overlap with the stage II activity of interim monitoring. However, an important distinction is that study staff are actively involved in stage I data analysis activities, while study investigators and staff are typically not privy to the findings generated in stage II activities that are related to items 3 to 5 above, because they involve study outcomes. *Only designated statisticians have access to the outcome data for interim analysis.* Interim analyses are typically presented to an independent Data and Safety Monitoring Board (DSMB), sometimes called a Data Monitoring Committee (DMC).

"Look and Learn": Trial Monitoring not Involving Outcome Measures

The "look and learn" component of interim monitoring of a trial is unrelated to the study outcome measures, and it is in the best interests of the trial to review these types of accruing data on a regular basis, and to consider corrective measures as needed. Enrollment reports are the most universal tool for monitoring trial progress. It is important to examine enrollment:

- By stage of recruitment (i.e., number screened, number eligible, number enrolled).
- By site, to determine highest and lowest recruiting sites, and to improve performance by sharing the recruitment approaches of the highest-enrolling sites with others.

- By actual versus expected for period to date, to assess whether target sample size can be achieved by planned end, or whether modifications to the trial timeline, number of participating sites, eligibility criteria, or recruitment approach are needed.
- By time period, to assess whether there are seasonal variations in recruitment or whether "trial fatigue" is occurring in an extended recruitment period.

Figure 5.1 shows a useful chart for trial enrollment that provides immediate visual impact, in addition to quantitative information that is not provided by a standard summary enrollment report. Due to the use of shading for time intervals since the last enrollment within a site, it is quickly evident which sites have had steady recruitment activity, and where activity has lagged. There is also information regarding the initiation date of each site, in the case of staggered entry into the trial. Lastly, the chart facilitates tracking of monthly enrollment, which is helpful for projections. This grid can be used for reporting in conjunction with a line graph of actual versus expected enrollment to track progress.

A summary of protocol compliance is also an important interim monitoring tool to assess the integrity of the trial. If the study cannot be executed as designed, study hypotheses cannot be examined as intended. Two types of violations are usually examined:

Site	January	February	March	April	May	June	July	August	September	October	November	December
01	3	1	3	3	3		1	1	1		3	1
02	3	1	2		1	2	1		1	1		
03		2	2	1	3	1				1		2
04	5	1	3	1			1				1	3
05				3	9	7	8	5	3	5	4	
06			1	3	1	1	2	4		3	1	1
07	2		2	1		3		2	2			
08	2	2	1	2								
09								3	5		1	1
10	2	3	2		4	5	3	2	1	2		3
Total	17	10	16	14	21	19	16	17	13	12	10	11

■ = time since last enrollment
▒ = time prior to site initiation

FIGURE 5.1 Example of a trial enrollment grid.

1. Eligibility violations—the identification of subjects who are found after enrollment to have been ineligible at the time of randomization.
2. Protocol violations—processes related to treatment administration and trial measurements that are not performed as specified. These events should be defined before trial start by specifications in the protocol, and each type of violation is typically classified as major or minor (with minor sometimes referred to as a deviation rather than violation). Examples of violations are incorrect delivery of an intervention and trial outcome measurements that are not made, or made out-of-window. Violations should be examined both overall as well as by site.

A high rate overall may suggest that retraining is needed for all participants, or that a particular aspect of the clinical protocol might need to be modified, because the timing or method of measurement is infeasible. In other instances, violations of a certain type are specific to a site and these can be remedied by working directly with site staff to increase awareness of and compliance with the recruitment and measurement protocol.

The "look and learn" component of interim monitoring by site staff and investigator is important because it provides information about whether the trial can be executed on time (and consequently, on budget), and executed as designed. If the trial is deemed infeasible with regard to either issue, two levels of action are typically considered:

1. Modification of trial design. Examples include modification of eligibility criteria to broaden the target population (as long as this does not lead to an inability to address the scientific question of interest or dilute the expected treatment effect, thus lowering power), or addition of more sites to increase capture of the target population as originally designed. Pinpointing how to modify eligibility criteria or recruitment procedures is facilitated by study flowcharts of what subgroups most often fail to meet eligibility criteria or who declines to consent.
2. Termination of the trial for failure to recruit or failure to be executed properly. This is an extreme measure, but it has both ethical and financial motivations. If the trial will be severely underpowered, it is considered unethical to knowingly enroll patients into a randomized study with the knowledge that their data will not be sufficient to answer the primary trial hypothesis. From a practical point of view, financial resources for research are nearly always limited, and despite an investment in trial development and implementation, if the trial will be underpowered or flawed in its delivery of the intervention or collection or measurement of outcomes, then it may not be sound or practical to commit additional resources to the study.

"Restricted Access Only": Trial Monitoring of Variance—Adaptive Design

Often despite best efforts to use accurate assumptions in sample size calculations, observed outcomes may not conform. A useful type of "restricted access only" monitoring is to estimate the variance of the primary outcome part of the way through the trial period, before accrual is completed. Statistical power decreases as variance increases. If the primary endpoint of the trial is a proportion, then the variance of the proportion increases as the proportion of subjects with the trial endpoint approaches 0.5. If the variance is found in interim analysis to be larger than that used for the original trial design, an increase in target sample size might be considered. Such modifications fall under the category of adaptive design.[1-4] It is important to note that *the observed treatment difference should not be used in decisions regarding modification of sample size.* However, it is acceptable to estimate the variance in a single treatment arm, typically the arm considered to be standard therapy, as the sample size calculation is often based on this arm, with sample size determined by utilizing a specified minimum clinically significant difference from the standard.

"Restricted Access Only": Formal Interim Trial Monitoring Procedures—Analysis of Outcomes

The remaining reasons for "restricted access only" interim monitoring are to assess safety and efficacy during the conduct of the trial. These analyses are, at appropriate time points, conducted by treatment arm, and are what most researchers think of as interim analysis. The choice of specific type of interim monitoring plan is made during the trial design period. There is a large literature on design and analysis methodology for examining trial outcomes by treatment group prior to the end of the trial.[5-7] The most common of these methods is called group sequential design, which is a class of approaches to compare treatments at one or more time points before trial end, with appropriate adjustment to the significance level of the multiple statistical tests conducted so that the pre-specified overall Type I error rate for the trial primary endpoint comparison is preserved. Conditional power calculations are another tool.[8]

With regard to efficacy, a trial may be stopped early because of a large observed treatment difference; or conversely, stopped due to futility—evidence that the null hypothesis will fail to be rejected and the trial will show no significant difference between treatment groups.[9] Regardless of the specific monitoring methodology employed, there are issues discussed below, that generally arise during formal interim monitoring of trial data and its presentation.

Aggregate Versus Treatment-Specific Interim Analyses

When is it appropriate to examine trial results by treatment arm? The importance of a prespecified interim analysis plan is paramount in this regard. Suppose a trial design specifies two equally spaced interim looks at the data over the course of a 4-year trial duration, and the Data and Safety Monitoring Board meets semiannually. There will be meetings at six interim time points, but only two with official "looks" at the data. At the meetings for which an interim look at the data by treatment arm is not scheduled, the outcomes measuring treatment *efficacy* should be presented in aggregate, that is, with both treatment arms combined. Outcomes measuring the *safety* of the interventions, however, are presented by treatment arm.

Presentation of efficacy outcomes in aggregate allows assessment of the overall event rate or mean outcome value for a study, and its associated variance, but prevents the trial from being subjected to additional looks that could alter the overall Type I error rate for the primary comparison. However, even when outcome data are presented in aggregate, information can be gleaned about the observed treatment difference. For example, if the overall event rate in a trial is lower than expected, it implies that there is less room for a treatment difference to be observed. *Therefore, study investigators should not view outcome data from interim analyses, even if presented in aggregate.*

Interim monitoring of safety outcomes is also an important responsibility of the DSMB. These outcomes *must* be provided by treatment arm, because adverse events experienced may be specific to the intervention. There are two reference points for evaluation of safety outcomes—comparison to historical rates of adverse events for a given intervention, and comparison of a new or investigative therapy to an existing standard used in the trial. If the adverse event rate for the nonstandard therapy is significantly higher than expected, there are several options:

- Modification of the interventional procedure to address the specific safety concern (e.g., decreasing the therapy intensity by reducing dose, duration, or both; alteration of surgical technique or perioperative treatment).
- Dropping the experimental arm showing unacceptable adverse event rates (if there are more than two such arms in the trial).
- Early termination of the trial (if there are only two arms in the trial).

With regard to the last option, one can also devise formal statistical rules for early stopping related to safety outcomes. When safety (inferiority) is considered from the start to be a high concern, the DSMB will typically recommend that the trial protocol specify a stopping rule for safety in addition to an early stopping rule for efficacy, with spending of the Type I error for the two aspects of monitoring being considered independent of each other.

Blinding of Treatment Arm in Interim Monitoring— A Controversial Topic

When interim analyses of study outcomes by treatment arm are presented to a monitoring board, the report can be blinded or unblinded. If blinded, then the treatment arms are assigned letter codes such as A and B, and the link to the specific arm is not revealed. In this setting, the same letter codes would be used across all interim reports, in order for the DSMB to follow patterns in the accruing data. The argument in favor of the practice of blinding is that the DSMB's decision on whether to stop a trial prematurely should be based on the size of the treatment effect and not its direction. Others, however, particularly in recent years, have argued that the DSMB should have all information at its disposal to make the most informed decision possible about safety as well as efficacy of an intervention. The pros and cons of these two approaches have been discussed at length.[10–12] A compromise approach is to prepare interim analysis reports with blinded treatment notation (A versus B), but to allow the statistician to reveal the link to DSMB members verbally upon request. An additional benefit of blinded presentation of trial results, even if the DSMB is made aware of the link, is that the notation prevents a breach of confidentiality of results should this report be inadvertently obtained by others.

Stage III

In stage III, final analysis, the benefits of ongoing data cleaning and quality review of the accruing data are realized. The analysis should follow the plan specified in the trial protocol, and examine the primary as well as secondary trial endpoints, for all subjects as well as for prespecified subgroups. Approaches to the final analyses are discussed below.

APPROACHES TO ANALYSIS

In this section, for simplicity but with no loss of generality, it is assumed that there are two treatments under study. Typically, the two treatments will be a new or unproven/experimental treatment versus a standard or (placebo) control.

Primary Analysis of Trial Endpoints

When a randomized clinical trial protocol is finalized, it contains a pre-specified analysis plan for the trial endpoints. The analysis plan should distinguish between the *primary and secondary analyses* of trial endpoints. The terms primary analysis and secondary analysis should not be confused with the type of trial outcome (primary outcome versus secondary outcome). The primary analysis plan specifies methods to be used for all trial endpoints and accommodates the specific features of the design, such as random treatment assignment. The findings from the primary analysis plan are nearly always those that determine whether the trial is "positive" or "negative" and are considered to deliver the main message of a trial when published. The secondary analysis of trial data may specify several approaches, alone or in combination, that address alternative interpretation of the data. This is sometimes necessary when the protocol is not executed exactly as designed. Secondary analyses may also utilize alternative statistical approaches for an endpoint. Typically, the goal of secondary analytic approaches is to confirm (or explain) the results of the primary analyses.

Intention to Treat (ITT)

For Phase III randomized clinical trials (and for some Phase II trials), the primary analysis plan for study outcomes is always according to the intention-to-treat principle. This principle means that trial subjects are retained in their assigned treatment group for the purpose of analysis, *regardless of actual treatment received.*

The purpose of intention-to-treat analysis is to minimize bias in the estimated treatment effect. Randomization is a powerful tool that ensures that any differences observed in trial outcomes are attributable to the assigned treatment and not to other factors, because the trial subjects will be similar with respect to all other factors. At the time of final analysis there is a temptation to reclassify patients into the "right" group, according to what treatment was actually received. However, the reclassification of a subject into the opposite treatment group corrupts the balance that is achieved by the randomization process. As an example, consider age, which is highly correlated with mortality. Randomization ensures that the subjects in the assigned treatment groups will, on average, be of similar age; therefore, any differences observed in treatment cannot be attributed to age. However, if the data of selected subjects are shifted into the opposite treatment group, and the reason for subjects receiving the opposite treatment is age-related, then the two groups composed from a non-intention-to-treat analysis may be unbalanced with respect to age. Therefore the mortality comparison will be biased; inference regarding a causal effect of treatment is no longer possible. Non-ITT as a secondary analysis is discussed below.

There is a tradeoff, of course—minimization of bias in the estimated treatment effect comes at the price of lower statistical power to detect a specified treatment effect conditional on sample size. *When subjects are retained in their assigned treatment group, the estimated treatment effect will be diluted inevitably towards the null hypothesis of no difference* (see Chapter 4 for a full discussion of dilution). However, lower statistical power is preferable to a biased treatment effect estimate, since the underlying reason for a randomized clinical trial is to make inferences about the efficacy of a treatment in the absence of influence from other factors. Of note as an exception, in a Phase II study, where the aim is to identify the most effective dose of a therapy to be used as a treatment arm in a later controlled trial, a non-ITT analysis is preferred and appropriate.

Impact of Dilution on Analysis
Treatment Crossovers

Because an intention-to-treat analysis is preferable for Phase III trials but will reflect dilution of treatment effect if crossover occurs, in the design phase of the trial it is important to estimate the crossover rate in each direction (A to B and B to A), and the effect size used in sample size calculations to ensure the desired level of power in the presence of the diluted (smaller) treatment effect (see Chapter 4). Accounting in advance for crossover will increase the required sample size. In the analysis phase, although the estimated treatment effect from the intention-to-treat analysis in the presence of crossover will be smaller than that achieved using a non-intent-to-treat analysis, the larger sample size accrued will increase precision correspondingly.

No Study Treatment Administered

What is the appropriate way to handle data when a randomized subject receives neither of the two treatments under study? One could argue that such a subject can provide no information about the relative efficacy of the two treatments under study. In this setting, it is considered acceptable by some trialists to remove the subject from the final primary analysis, assuming that the following condition is met: *the reason for receiving no study treatment is completely independent of the treatment assignment itself.*[13] If this independence is present, then the subjects excluded (from either treatment group) will be random with respect to

> **EXAMPLE OF LEGITIMATE REMOVAL OF SUBJECTS FROM ANALYSIS**
>
> The Pediatric Heart Network Single Ventricle Reconstruction trial randomly assigns infants who are born with one rather than two functional ventricles to receive one of two surgical techniques shortly after birth. The primary outcome is death or cardiac transplantation at 1 year.
>
> A small number of these infants do not undergo the surgery, and therefore their outcome does not contribute any information regarding the relative efficacy of technique A versus technique B. These infants typically do not undergo the surgery either because of rapid clinical decline after birth or misdiagnosis of the anatomic condition that leads to an alternative repair being appropriate.
>
> In either instance, the reason for not receiving assigned treatment is unrelated to the treatment assignment itself, and their outcomes are not of interest because they received neither surgical technique. It is therefore possible to conclude that their exclusion from either treatment group is random, and no bias is introduced by exclusion of such subjects from the primary trial analysis.

their underlying characteristics. Therefore the composition of the two treatment groups after exclusion of such subjects in theory remains balanced with regard to both measured and unmeasured patient and disease characteristics, and no bias is introduced into the treatment effect estimate.

Secondary Analysis of Trial Endpoints

Secondary analysis approaches are also important to specify in advance in the trial protocol, rather than after trial results have been preliminarily examined. Three of the most common types of secondary analysis are (i) approaches that account for protocol noncompliance, (ii) covariate-adjusted analyses, and (iii) analytic techniques for an endpoint that provide additional information on treatment efficacy.

Protocol Noncompliance

Protocol noncompliance typically takes two forms: (i) failure to deliver the assigned treatment as specified by the protocol or (ii) enrollment of a subject into the trial who is later determined to have been ineligible at the time of randomization.

Failure to Deliver the Treatment as Specified A non-ITT analysis is usually specified as a secondary analysis. This is achieved by classifying subjects according to the treatment actually received. In many instances, this is clear-cut and the data for a subject are analyzed as if belonging to the treatment group to which the subject has crossed over. In such an analysis, treatment remains a categorical variable. The goal is to determine the size of the treatment effect without dilution from subjects who did not receive an assigned treatment or were not compliant with the treatment protocol, as discussed earlier. Heavy caution is required in the interpretation of such an analysis given the likely bias in comparing treatment groups. The preferred outcome is to demonstrate results consistent with the primary analysis results. This consistency strengthens the results of the trial. Lack of consistency may detract from trial results if not well explained.

It should also be noted that when classifying subjects according to dose received, some subjects may not remain in the analysis. If the total dose received is below a threshold defined as "treated," then the subject may belong in neither treatment group. For example, perhaps "compliant" in an active drug versus placebo trial is defined as receiving 85% of total dose expected (for the placebo group, this definition implies that the subject received no active drug at least 85% of the time). Then if a subject assigned to the drug group does not meet this definition, but did receive more than 15% of total dose expected, then his or her data would be excluded from both groups because it does not meet the drug definition of compliant (Table 5.1). In the other extreme, if the subject was assigned to the active drug and received no more than 15% of total dose expected, his or her data would be included in the placebo group analyses. If total dose received was between 15% and 85%, the data would be excluded from the non-ITT analysis.

If estimation of the dose–response relationship is of interest, then treatment may take the form of a continuous measure rather than a categorical indicator for treatment received. Such a measure might be the percentage of total dose expected, or the actual total dose received adjusted for body size. Regression analysis of outcome on dose would then be applied, rather than a comparison of outcome for two distinct groups. Such an analysis would also permit exploration of nonlinear relationships between dose and outcome.

Table 5.1 — Classification of Subjects According to Treatment Received Using an 85% Threshold

% of Total *Expected* Dose Received	Classify Subjects Into: Active Treatment	Placebo/Control
Assigned to Placebo		
<15%[a]	X	
15–84%	Exclude	Exclude
≥85%		X
Assigned to Active Treatment		
<15%[b]		X
15–84%	Exclude	Exclude
≥85%	X	

[a] Assumes crossover to active drug if placebo not received as expected.
[b] Assumes no other nontrial clinical treatments administered.

Inclusion of Ineligible Subjects How should one handle ineligible randomized subjects? Despite careful screening of potential study subjects and documentation of their clinical and demographic characteristics, it is sometimes unavoidable that the following sequence of events occurs: a patient is considered eligible based on all information on hand at the time, provides informed consent, and is randomized, but at a later date is determined to have been ineligible at the time of randomization. Typically, a secondary analysis of all trial endpoints is specified in the protocol to exclude such subjects. Because in some instances the subject who is deemed ineligible post-randomization may not represent the patient population of interest, one might consider whether his or her data should be excluded from even primary analysis of study endpoints. There are two types of ineligible patients:

1. Those who do not have the condition of interest that is under study.
2. Those who have the condition of interest, but its severity may not match trial eligibility criteria.

The response to treatment of patients in the first scenario may not be relevant because they do not have the condition under study. As an example, in the Pediatric Heart Network Kawasaki Disease Trial of Pulsed Steroid Therapy, a patient was randomized who was determined later to have not Kawasaki disease but Ebstein-Barr virus. In the SHOCK trial, a patient was randomized who had the clinical signs and symptoms of cardiogenic shock, but after randomization when an echocardiogram was performed, it was evident that the dramatic drop in blood pressure and systemic hypoperfusion was due to an aortic dissection. These patients do not have the diagnosis of interest. It should be noted that ineligible but randomized patients are equally likely to be assigned to either treatment group, and therefore their response does not lead to a biased estimate of treatment effect.

It is important to note that, under many conditions, inclusion of these subjects in primary analysis provides *face validity to the trial*. In the real world, patients also receive treatment based on knowledge of their condition at presentation, and this may include patients who are misdiagnosed as well as patients whose severity of disease may differ from initial assessment. By inclusion of all randomized subjects in the primary analysis regardless of eligibility, the estimate of treatment efficacy reflects the "real-world" public health impact of the therapy. A secondary analysis of trial outcomes, with ineligible subjects excluded, provides an estimate of treatment efficacy in its purest form. This secondary analysis is of particular interest when the primary result is negative and the proportion of ineligible subjects is high enough to affect the primary trial results. Here, the result of interest is whether the treatment has benefit if applied only to the target population?

Covariate-Adjusted Analysis

In addition to protocol noncompliance, another type of secondary analysis of trial endpoints often specified in a trial protocol is a covariate-adjusted treatment group comparison. Due to the power of randomization, an unadjusted primary analysis of trial data is usually specified to report the main trial result. *With sufficiently large sample size, randomization ensures treatment arms are balanced with regard to baseline factors, both measured and unmeasured, and therefore the unadjusted comparison provides an unbiased estimate of treatment effect.* However, the mean value (for example, baseline age), or prevalence (for example, proportion of males), of one or more characteristics may be found at the end of the trial to be different for the two treatment arms. Although any difference in baseline characteristics must be due to chance if randomization is working properly, the imbalance may lead to a biased estimate of treatment effect if the observed imbalance is with respect to a factor or measurement that is related to study outcome. Specification of a secondary covariate-adjusted regression analysis of trial outcomes allows for statistical correction of such observed imbalances to provide an unbiased treatment effect estimate. The estimated mean treatment group difference $\overline{Y}_1 - \overline{Y}_2$ in the presence of a covariate X can be expressed as:

$$\overline{Y}_1 - \overline{Y}_2 = \beta_1 + \beta_2(\overline{X}_1 - \overline{X}_2)$$

where β_1 is the unadjusted treatment effect estimate, β_2 is the effect estimate for the covariate, and $\overline{X}_1$ and $\overline{X}_2$ are the mean values of the covariate in treatment groups 1 and 2, respectively. *The term $b_2(\overline{X}_1 - \overline{X}_2)$ is the potential size of the bias.* If the two treatment arms are not balanced with respect to X, then $\overline{X}_1 - \overline{X}_2$ is nonzero. If X is related to study outcome, then β_2 is nonzero. Of note, as stated above, if there is imbalance in X but β_2 is zero (i.e., no association between a baseline factor and study outcome), then the unadjusted treatment effect estimate remains unbiased.

Adjustment for imbalances in baseline characteristics not only reduces bias but can increase precision of the treatment effect, particularly when linear regression is the adjustment method. The standard error of the covariate-adjusted treatment effect comparison will be reduced when the covariate is related to outcome, because the variation in the outcome that can be explained by the covariate more than compensates for the loss of a degree of freedom in the residual error term. *For this reason, a covariate-adjusted comparison of treatment effect is desirable as a prespecified secondary analysis even when no imbalances by treatment arm exist.* Selection of the adjustment factors is usually specified *a priori* at the design stage, based on current known correlates of the study outcome. Indeed, the most powerful treatment effect comparison may be a covariate-adjusted one, and with proper advance specification such a comparison may even be appropriate as the primary analysis for the trial.

Alternative Statistical Approaches

A final type of secondary analysis does not deal with modification of the treatment classification, the subjects to be included, or with the completeness of the data, but rather with how to maximize information from a trial endpoint and enhance interpretation. Simply put, there may be more than one way to analyze an endpoint. One method will be considered primary, but alternative methods may also be appropriate and informative. For example, if length of hospital stay is the trial outcome, one might specify the primary analysis to be a comparison of log-transformed mean values from the two treatment groups. However, the pattern of discharges may also be relevant and time-to-discharge analysis using Kaplan-Meier curves and a logrank test might be specified as a secondary analysis of the same endpoint. In this example, one might find that mean log-transformed length of stay does not vary by treatment group, but perhaps the hazard functions of time-to-discharge vary, and hypotheses regarding the shape of this hazard function can be evaluated using a time-to-event analysis.

Subgroup Analyses

We have discussed analysis approaches with the aim of estimating overall treatment effect. However, an important component of nearly all statistical analysis plans is the analysis of patient subgroups. To be valid, these analyses must:

- Have patient subgroup *definitions prespecified* in the trial protocol.
- Have subgroup definitions based on factors that are *known at baseline*.
- Identify significant differential treatment effects by subgroup using a *test of interaction*, not within-subgroup treatment comparisons.

Subgroup analyses can be of particular interest when the overall trial result is negative. This result may be masking a treatment effect that truly exists for a patient subgroup. If such an effect exists, it can result in benefit to selected patients and the viability of a new treatment for a targeted population. However, hypotheses about subgroups should be generated during trial design and included in the protocol. If a very large number of subgroups are examined, a significant result may occur due to chance.

Even in the best of circumstances, subgroup analyses must be interpreted with caution. The requirement that the subgroup definition be based on a factor or condition that is known at baseline has both a practical and scientific rationale. If the subgroup factor cannot be known at baseline, then one cannot identify the patients at diagnosis or presentation who are most likely to benefit and who should therefore receive the treatment. From a scientific perspective, the power of a randomized trial is that differences in outcome can be attributed to the treatment because all other patient characteristics are similar in the treatment groups, due to randomization. *However, when the treatment effects are examined within subgroup, particularly a subgroup that was not a stratification factor in the randomization scheme, there is no guarantee that the characteristics of the patients in the two treatment arms within a subgroup will be balanced.* This means that the finding of a significant treatment effect within a patient subgroup could be due to a factor other than the treatment.

A positive subgroup finding is only valid if the treatment effect is compared to that estimated for the remainder of the sample; that is, *a treatment arm by subgroup factor interaction test must be employed using all the trial data.*[14] Although it is not uncommon for many trial reports to declare subgroup findings based on a simple within-subgroup comparison of treatment groups, this approach is flawed, typically overestimating significance.[15] Suppose, for example, the subgroup factor is presence versus absence of diabetes at randomization. The hypothesis that must be tested is not whether outcome in treatment A versus treatment B is significantly different within the subgroup of diabetic patients. The analysis must demonstrate that the treatment effect for diabetics, however measured, differs significantly from the treatment effect observed for nondiabetics. Only if the test of this interaction is statistically significant is it appropriate to then test whether the within-subgroup treatment effects differ from the null hypothesis. In the absence of interaction, it is inappropriate to conduct a two-group comparison in a particular patient subgroup to look for treatment effectiveness.

Figure 5.2 shows a typical method for graphical display of subgroup findings. Important features to include are the sample size of each subgroup, the point estimate of treatment effect (optionally, some figures make the size of the point estimate plotting symbol proportional to subgroup sample size), the interaction p-value, x-axis notation regarding the directionality of effect, and error bars to indicate variability of the estimate (95% confidence limits). In this figure, the overall SHOCK trial point estimate for treatment efficacy (relative risk for 30-day mortality) is shown, along with the effect estimates by subgroup.[16] We can see that the interaction p-value is significant for age group and for the presence versus absence of prior myocardial infarction. For age, the interaction ($p = 0.02$) exists because emergency revascularization is of benefit for patients under age 75 years, but there is no significant treatment effect in patients aged ≥75 years. Of note, later analyses also demonstrated that within the elderly subgroup, a key prognostic factor (left ventricular ejection fraction) was unbalanced by treatment group, accounting in part for the lack of benefit of emergency revascularization in this subgroup—the possibility of imbalances in important baseline characteristics by treatment within subgroup must always be kept in mind as an explanatory factor for subgroup findings. There is no differential treatment effect according to diabetes or gender. For gender, it is important to note that although the 95% confidence interval for the relative risk does not include one for the male subgroup and does include one for the

Subgroup	N		Interaction p
All Subjects			
Age <75 years	246		.01
Age ≥75 years	56		
Males	205		.15
Females	97		
Prior MI	98		.57
No Prior MI	204		
Diabetes	92		.02
No Diabetes	204		

Relative Risk

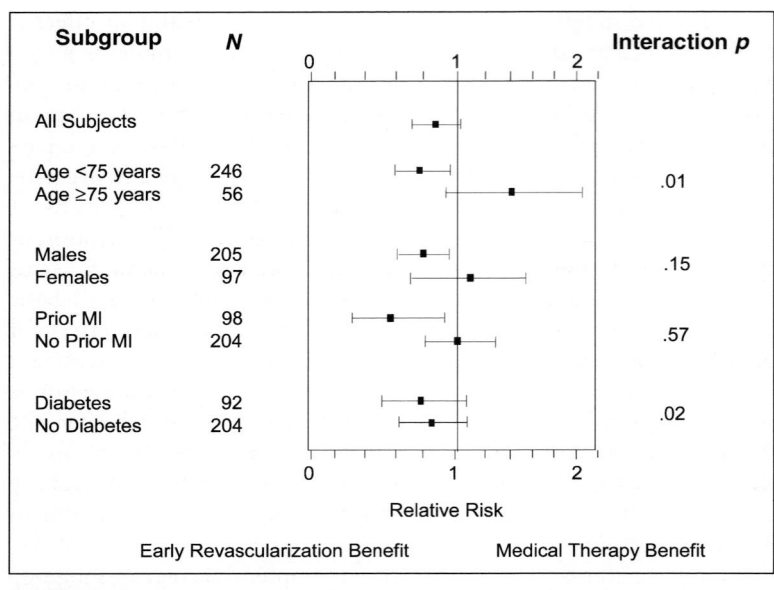

Early Revascularization Benefit — Medical Therapy Benefit

FIGURE 5.2 A typical method for graphical display of subgroup findings.

female subgroup, these two relative risks (0.75 versus 1.06) do not differ sufficiently for the gender by treatment group interaction to be significant. In this instance, we conclude that the overall trial risk reduction of 17% (relative risk 0.83) attributable to emergency revascularization is applicable to all subjects, regardless of gender.

Missing Data

In any research study, investigators must contend with a variety of sources of missing data:

- Subjects may be lost through death, refusal to participate further, movement to new locations, missed interim visits, or refusal of a particular procedure.
- Specimen volumes may not be sufficient for all planned laboratory tests, diagnostic equipment may malfunction, or specimens may be mishandled.
- Imaging studies may be of poor quality and therefore uninterpretable; even among interpretable images, selected quantitative measures may not be available.

Missing at Random or Not?
The effect of missing data on the results of a trial depends upon whether the data are missing at random. If the probability that observations are obtained or missed is unrelated to the values of the observations, then the data are missing at random. If, however, patients with a more severe course of disease are more likely to miss study visits, for example, then the missing data are unlikely to be missing at random. Of note in the setting of a time-to-event trial outcome, the term for nonrandom missingness is *informative censoring*.[17] If data are missing at random, then the power of the study to identify the stated treatment effect will be reduced due to the smaller sample size of a complete case analysis. If, however, the missing data are not missing at random, then the estimated treatment effect may be biased. At a minimum, the result can be expressed only as a conditional finding. Chapter 9 provides an excellent discussion of the impact of loss to follow-up.

The Special Case of Quality-of-Life Outcomes
A conditional analysis may be perfectly appropriate and clinically relevant, for example, if a trial secondary endpoint is quality of life (QOL) in a study where mortality is the primary endpoint, and QOL measures will be completed only for those subjects still alive at the visit for which QOL assessment is required. Therefore, the mean QOL scores are conditional on being alive at that time point, and are easily interpretable. However, if there are QOL measurements missing for any other reason, such as failure to return for a study visit because of an improved (or worsened) clinical state, then this type of nonrandom missingness renders effect estimates that do not reflect the state of all survivors.

To Impute or Not?
There is a large body of statistical literature on methodology for missing data analysis[18] and the required assumptions. These include:

- Last-observation carried forward.
- Mean imputation.
- Worst case imputation.
- Multiple imputation.

There are tradeoffs in the selection of these methods with regard to both statistical properties as well as practical issues of implementation and interpretation. Regardless of which method is chosen, a sensitivity analysis for final trial results is usually desirable. If we can demonstrate that the trial has the same magnitude of treatment effect, regardless of

> **THINGS TO REMEMBER FOR ANALYSIS**
> - Both primary and secondary analytic approaches should be pre-specified for all trial endpoints.
> - Randomization is a powerful tool that ensures no bias, and is the underpinning of an ITT analysis.
> - Dilution of treatment effects reduces power, but a potentially more powerful non-ITT analysis has unknown biases that can lead to incorrect inferences.
> - To avoid bias when excluding subjects who received neither study treatment, the reason for not receiving study treatment must be independent of the treatment assignment.
> - Covariate adjustment removes bias caused by imbalance in baseline characteristics *and* can increase precision.
> - In the best of all possible analyses, data that are not collected should be missing at random; but they seldom are.

whether complete case analysis or an analysis involving some form of imputation has been utilized, then the trial findings will be considered robust.

ANALYTIC METHODS

This section will not attempt to construct a statistical textbook of methods, which is covered by numerous texts already (see the Recommended Reading suggestions at the end of the chapter). It will describe the main approaches for continuous, categorical, and censored outcomes, as well as briefly discuss p-values, confidence intervals, and post-hoc power analyses.

There are three major types of outcome data:

1. Continuous
2. Categorical
3. Time-to-event, with possible censoring

Continuous Outcomes

When the outcome is continuous, the analytic method ranges from the simplest two-group unadjusted comparison by t-test or Wilcoxon rank sum test, to mixed model regression for longitudinal outcomes, and analysis of variance for cluster and factorial designs, including random effects models for crossover designs.

Categorical Outcomes

When the outcome is categorical, analytic methods include Fisher exact or chi-square test for a two-group comparison of a 2 × 2 table, logistic regression for binary outcomes with baseline or other covariate adjustment, and cumulative logistic or multinomial logistic regression for ordered and nonordered multiple-category outcomes. If an outcome is ordered but the assumption of proportional odds does not hold, then in this instance also multinomial regression is employed.

If multiple occurrences of a primary outcome dichotomous event are possible per subject, then Poisson regression is used. Examples include analysis of incidence of stroke or MI, or analysis of the number of acute painful crises in sickle-cell disease. In both instances, a subject may experience the event more than once.

Time-to-Event Outcomes

When the outcome is time to event, such as time to death or time to discharge, then a two-group or multiple-group unadjusted comparison is conducted using a test from the family of weighted score tests. The most common of these is the logrank test, where all test statistic weights are one. Another test from this class that is often used is the Gehan-Wilcoxon test,[19] which weights each component of the statistic according to number of subjects at risk at each observed failure time; thus the test statistic is influenced most by differences between groups that occur early. Cox proportional hazards regression[20] is employed when an adjusted group comparison is required, or to accommodate multiple events per subject. Parametric models for time-to-event outcomes are also possible (e.g., Weibull), but are less common in clinical settings.

Time-to-event outcomes can include censored observations. Censoring occurs particularly in trials where the length of follow-up is not uniform across subjects due to staggered entry over time and a fixed trial end date. Typically, in clinical studies, if censoring is present, it is right-censored—that is, the event of interest is not observed by trial end. All of the methods described above accommodate censored observations. Censoring of observations is also used for analysis of competing risks—for example, when death and heart transplantation are both possible outcomes that affect the cumulative incidence function for one or more of the events of interest.[21]

Statistical methods that account for both the time to event and the possibility of multiple events per subject fall into the class of Cox regression models for multivariate failure times, which are derived from counting process theory.[22,23] Classical survival analysis assumes that all failure times are independent. The multivariate failure time approach constructs adjustments to the parameter estimates (e.g., the hazard ratio) to account for the correlated nature of the events that occur in clusters (e.g., multiple events arising from one subject). The multivariate failure time approach may also be used for studies where there may be only one event per subject, but the subjects in the trial are not all independent, such as family members.

REPORTING OF RESULTS

Regardless of the type of study outcome or the analysis method employed, the same principles are applied to reporting. It is important to relay:

1. The size of the estimated treatment effect.
2. The variance associated with the estimated treatment effect.
3. The result of significance testing, and its interpretation.

Reporting Magnitude of Effect and Its Variance

To convey the results of a randomized trial, it is important to provide an estimate of the *magnitude* of the treatment effect as well as its associated *variance*. We want to know how much impact the intervention had on outcome, and whether the difference observed between treatments is within expected limits of natural variation. These pieces of information form the basis for a statistical test or construction of a confidence interval. The statistical test provides a *p-value* on which to base inferences regarding treatment efficacy and safety. Alternatively, a confidence interval for the treatment effect estimate can be formed, particularly for reporting results of an equivalence or noninferiority trial. Table 5.2 outlines the types of treatment effect estimates used according to the type of outcome.

Continuous Outcomes

For a continuous outcome, the most common estimate of treatment effect is the mean difference $\overline{Y}_1 - \overline{Y}_2$ between groups. Examples of outcomes where the mean difference would be used to relay the magnitude of treatment effect include blood pressure, weight-for-age z-score in children, or a quality of life score. If the mean difference is not zero, we

Table 5.2 Summary of Outcome Data Type and Treatment Effect Estimate

Outcome	Effect Estimate	Treatment Difference May Exist If
Continuous	Mean difference $\bar{Y}_1 - \bar{Y}_2$	$\bar{Y}_1 - \bar{Y}_2 \neq 0$
	Median difference $m_1 - m_2$	$m_1 - m_2 \neq 0$
Categorical	Rate Difference $p_1 - p_2$	$p_1 - p_2 \neq 0$
	Odds ratio $(OR = [p_1/(1-p_1)]/[p_2/(1-p_2)])$	$OR \neq 1$
	Relative risk $(RR = p_1/p_2)$	$RR \neq 1$
Time-to-event	Hazard ratio (HR)	$HR \neq 1$
	Incidence rate (IR) difference	$IR_1 - IR_2 \neq 0$

need to know whether the size of the difference is likely to have occurred by chance or whether the difference is so large that it is attributable to another factor. If sufficiently large, as determined by the statistical test conducted, the difference is attributed to the intervention, due to the randomized design.

Variability in the mean outcome from each group is expressed using the standard error of the mean, which is $s/\sqrt{n}$, where s is the standard deviation (person-to-person variation). The standard error of the mean decreases as the sample size n increases, proportional to the square root of n. The *standard error of the mean difference* between two treatment groups is $\sqrt{(s_1^2/n_1 + s_2^2/n_2)}$. The magnitude of the treatment difference is evaluated with respect to the standard error, which serves as the denominator of the hypothesis test for no treatment difference. When forming a confidence interval for the mean treatment difference, the standard error of the mean difference determines the width of the confidence interval, which will be narrower as the standard deviation becomes smaller and as the sample size becomes larger. The 95% confidence interval for the mean difference is $\bar{Y}_1 - \bar{Y}_2 \pm \sqrt{(s_1^2/n_1 + s_2^2/n_2)}$. The interpretation of the 95% confidence interval is that one can be 95% certain that the interval constructed contains the true treatment difference. Therefore, if the confidence interval for the true mean difference between groups contains zero, there is insufficient evidence to claim that the two treatments under study differ.

Categorical Outcomes

For a dichotomous outcome such as death by 1 year, the size of the treatment effect can be characterized in absolute or relative terms. The *absolute* rate difference $p_1 - p_2$, where p_1 and p_2 are the mortality rates in the two trial arms, is often of interest because the size of the absolute difference has clinical relevance, representing the number of lives saved per 100 patients. This measure is also called the absolute risk reduction. A drawback, however, is that a 3% improvement in mortality is important when the expected rate is, say, 6%; however, a 3% improvement may not be clinically significant when the expected event rate is 60%. The *relative difference* is of interest to report because it provides a measure of treatment effect that is independent of the underlying rates, allowing it to be compared across studies and across subgroup analyses. The odds ratio and relative risk (RR) are both relative measures of treatment effect, and are similar to each other when the event rate is very low. If the odds ratio or relative risk is far from 1, then the two treatments differ. The relative risk reduction, defined as $100\% \times (1 - RR)$, is another measure commonly reported.

Example Suppose that a trial of drug-eluting versus bare metal stents yields composite 1-year myocardial infarction/death rates of 5% versus 8% (Table 5.3). The rate difference is 0.03, and the odds ratio and relative risk are very similar (0.645 versus 0.625) because the event rates are low. The relative risk reduction is $100 \times (1 - 0.625) = 37.5\%$; in other words, the mortality rate of 5% is 37.5% lower than the 8% rate in the other arm. In another trial, suppose event rates are 25% versus 40%. The relative risk reduction is 37.5% in this example as well, but

Table 5.3 Choosing the Appropriate Measure of a Difference Between Rates or Proportions

Measure	Trial 1	Trial 2
p_1 vs. p_2	0.05 vs. 0.08	0.25 vs. 0.40
Rate difference	0.03	0.15
Odds ratio	0.645	0.500
Relative risk	0.625	0.625
Relative risk reduction	37.5%	37.5%

the absolute rate difference is 0.15. In addition, the odds ratio (0.50) is not as similar to the relative risk (0.625) because the event rates are farther from zero.

Time-to-Event Outcomes

In many trials, the length of follow-up time per subject varies because the first patient enrolled is followed until the last patient enrolled completes some minimum desired length of follow-up. For example, 2 years may be required to accrue the target sample size, and a minimum of 3 years of follow-up may be desired on each subject. Therefore, assuming a uniform rate of enrollment, the average follow-up time is 4 years, with a range from 3 to 5 years per subject. If the primary outcome measure for the trial encompasses all available follow-up to maximize power, then the primary result for trial reporting is typically a hazard ratio obtained from Cox proportional hazards regression, with simultaneous presentation of the treatment-specific time-to-event curves. Of note, the logrank test *p*-value is equivalent in large samples to that from the Cox proportional hazards score test for the null hypothesis that the hazard ratio is equal to 1. To enhance interpretability of the hazard ratio that is estimated based on all available follow-up, pointwise estimates (e.g., survival at 1, 3, 5 years) are usually provided as ancillary information to facilitate interpretation of the hazard ratio and its associated confidence interval and *p*-value. In other instances, a pointwise estimate may instead be specified as the primary endpoint despite the variable follow-up. In this setting, the pointwise estimate is derived from the overall survival distribution, but may be a less powerful comparison of treatment groups.

When multiple events of the same type can occur for each subject, a loss of information can occur if only the first event is used in analysis. To account for all events per subject, an incidence rate for each treatment arm is presented (number of events/total follow-up time), and the treatment effect is characterized by the incidence rate difference when Poisson regression is used, and by a hazard ratio when multivariate failure time modeling is used.

Reporting and Interpretation of *p*-Values

Irrespective of the type of trial outcome and the method employed to analyze it, the summary result of a statistical hypothesis test is the *p-value*. The *p*-value reflects the probability that the result observed could have occurred by chance if the null hypothesis is true, that is, if treatment truly has no association with outcome. If the *p*-value is smaller than a prespecified level, then the trial result is considered positive. Usually, the prespecified significance level is 0.05. If the treatment difference observed in the trial is so large that there is less than a 5% probability that it could occur when there is no true difference between treatments, then the null hypothesis is rejected, and we conclude that the intervention has an impact on outcome.

Other Choices of Significance Level
In certain instances, the prespecified significance level may be lower than 0.05, such as when:

- It is desirable to have a Type I error rate smaller than 0.05; that is, to minimize the likelihood of concluding that there is a treatment effect when one truly does not exist.
- There is an interim monitoring plan that requires adjustment (reduction) of the significance level of the final treatment group comparison in order for the overall Type I error of 0.05 to be maintained.
- There are numerous trial outcomes and one wishes to control for the possibility that a significant finding might occur by chance (although some argue that adjustment for multiple outcomes to control Type I error merely increases Type II error).[24]

What Is a "Positive Trial"?
It should be noted that most Phase III randomized trials comprised both a primary and multiple secondary endpoints, and the consistency of the results across the entire set of endpoints often provides the best picture of whether a treatment is effective. Although the p-value from statistical testing of the primary endpoint alone is often considered to be the defining factor as to whether a trial is positive or negative, it is important to report all trial endpoint results for consideration by others. Significant resources are expended for the conduct of a trial, and all aspects should be considered before reaching a conclusion about whether a treatment is safe and effective. The secondary endpoint results may suggest the mechanism of action for a treatment effect, or if the secondary outcome findings are inconsistent with those of the primary outcome, they may indicate that further study is needed or that a different mechanism of action is at play.

Post-Hoc Power Analysis
Often after a trial is conducted, particularly if no significant difference in outcome was found between treatment groups, there is interest in retrospectively calculating the power of the study to have detected the difference

observed given sample size accrued. However, power is a characteristic tied to a specific study design, and not to a single experiment that has already been conducted. If the null hypothesis was not rejected, then the power is zero. Power should be calculated at the time of study design for the minimum clinically important difference; the power to detect an observed smaller difference is irrelevant if the minimum clinically important difference was stated accurately. If the study has already been conducted and no significant difference was found, then by definition the power to detect the observed effect is low. To best gain information on the true treatment difference, it is recommended that a confidence interval be constructed from the study data. This interval will inform as to the range in which the true treatment difference lies. Levine and Ensom[25] provide a discussion of the pitfalls of post-hoc power analysis, as do others.[26,27]

SUMMARY

This chapter provides guidance for the analysis of data from randomized clinical trials. Analysis of trial data can and should occur at all stages of a study. The goal of some analyses is to monitor and improve trial conduct, and these findings should be shared with all involved in the study. Other interim analyses involving treatment group comparisons need to be conducted only according to a prespecified plan, and viewed by a restricted set of individuals charged with monitoring the safety and efficacy of study treatments.

Most randomized trials are resource-intensive with regard to the number and type of endpoints. Much emphasis is placed on the determination of a trial as "positive" or "negative." However, a broader view that encompasses interpretation of secondary endpoints to complement the primary outcome result is prudent to arrive at a final message regarding treatment efficacy. Related to this goal, both primary and secondary analyses of all endpoints are recommended. If consistency between the primary (unadjusted, full data) and secondary (adjusted or selected subjects) analyses is present, then the trial findings are much more robust.

Regardless of type of design, clear reporting of results is important and allows the reader to directly assess the message of the trial. A measure of the magnitude of treatment effect, in conjunction with its associated variance, is valuable for clinical interpretation of findings as well as for formal hypothesis testing or construction of a confidence interval to determine the range in which the true treatment difference most likely lies. A variety of simple and sophisticated statistical methodologies exist for analysis of trial data. As long as the integrity of the trial design is maintained, all approaches will contribute to a better understanding of the treatment under study.

REFERENCES

1. Shih WJ, Gould LA. Re-evaluating design specifications of longitudinal clinical trial without unblinding when the key response is rate of change. *Stat Med.* 1995;14:2239–2248.
2. Chow SC, Chang M. *Adaptive Design Methods in Clinical Trials.* Boca Raton: CRC Press; 2006.
3. Wittes J. On changing a long-term clinical trial midstream. *Stat Med.* 2002;27:2789–2795.
4. Zucker DM, Denne J. Sample-size redetermination for repeated measures studies. *Biometrics.* 2002;58:548–549.
5. DeMets D. Stopping guidelines vs. stopping rules: A practitioner's point of view. *Commun Stat Theory Methods.* 1984;13:2395–2417.
6. Fleming TR, O'Brien PC. A multiple testing procedure for clinical trials. *Biometrics.* 1979;35:549–556.
7. Pocock SJ. When to stop a clinical trial. *BMJ.* 1992;305:235–240.
8. Lan KK, Wittes J. The B-value: a tool for monitoring data. *Biometrics.* 1988;44:579–585.
9. Pampallona S, Tsiatis AA. Group sequential designs for one-sided and two-sided hypothesis testing with provision for early stopping in favor of the null hypothesis. *J Statist Plan Inf.* 1994;42:19–35.
10. Day SJ, Altman DG. Blinding in clinical trials and other studies. *BMJ.* 2000;321:504.
11. Boutron I, Estellat C, Guittet L, et al. Methods of blinding in reports of randomized controlled trials assessing pharmacologic treatments: a systematic review. *PLoS Med.* 2006;3:e425.
12. Shultz KF. Assessing allocation concealment and blinding in randomized controlled trials: why bother? *Evid-Based Med.* 2000;5:36–38.
13. International Conference on Harmonisation, Section E9. Statistical principles for clinical trials, November 2005. http://www.ich.org/cache/compo/475-272-1.html.
14. Gail M, Simon R. Testing for qualitative interactions between patient effects and patient subsets. *Biometrics.* 1985;41:361–372.
15. Assmann S, Pocock S, Enos L, et al. Subgroup analysis and other (mis)uses of baseline data in clinical trials. *Lancet.* 2000;355:1064–1069.
16. Hochman JS, Sleeper LA, Webb JG, et al. Early revascularization in acute myocardial infarction complicated by cardiogenic shock. *N Engl J Med* 1999;341:625–634.
17. Wu M, Carroll R. Estimation and comparison of changes in the presence of informative right censoring by modeling the censoring process. *Biometrics.* 1988;44:175–188.

18. Rubin DB. Inference and missing data. *Biometrika.* 1976;63:581–592.
19. Gehan EA. A generalized two-sample Wilcoxon test for doubly censored data. *Biometrika.* 1965;52:650–652.
20. Cox D. Regression models and life tables (with discussion). *J R Stat Soc B.* 1972;34:187–220.
21. Tai B, Machin D, White I, et al. Competing risks analysis of patients with osteosarcoma: a comparison of four different approaches. *Stat Med.* 2001;20: 661–684.
22. Andersen PK, Gill RD. Cox's regression model for counting processes: a large sample study. *Ann Stat.* 1982;10:1100–1120.
23. Lin DY. Cox regression analysis of multivariate failure time data: the marginal approach. *Stat Med.* 1994;13:2233–2247.
24. Feise RJ. Do multiple outcome measures require *p*-value adjustment? *BMC Med Res Methodol.* 2002;2:8.
25. Levine M, Ensom MHH. Post hoc power analysis: an idea whose time has passed. *Pharmacotherapy.* 2001;21:405–409.
26. Hoening JM, Heisey DM. The abuse of power: the pervasive fallacy of power calulations for data analysis. *Am Statistician.* 2001;55:19–24.
27. Goodman SN, Berlin JA. The use of predicted confidence intervals when planning experiments and the misuse of power when interpreting the results. *Ann Int Med.* 1994;121:200–206.

RECOMMENDED READING

Alpert PS. Tutorial in biostatistics: longitudinal data analysis (repeated measures) in clinical trials. *Stat Med.* 1999;18:1707–1732.
Dawson-Saunders B, Trapp RG. *Basic and Clinical Biostatistics.* Norwalk, CT: Appleton & Lange; 1990.
Fitzmaurice GM, Laird NM, Ware JH. *Applied Longitudinal Analysis.* Hoboken, NJ: Wiley; 2004.
Jennison C, Turnbull BW. *Group Sequential Methods with Applications to Clinical Trials.* Boca Raton: Chapman & Hall/CRC; 2000.
Lee ET, Wang JW. *Statistical Methods for Survival Data Analysis.* 3rd ed. New York: Wiley; 2003.
Little RJA, Rubin D. *Missing Data. Statistical Analysis with Missing Data.* 2nd ed. New York: Wiley; 2002.
Meinert CL. *Clinical Trials: Design, Conduct, and Analysis.* New York: Oxford University Press; 1986.
Piantadosi S. *Clinical Trials: A Methodologic Perspective.* New York: Wiley; 1997.
Rosner B. *Fundamentals of Biostatistics.* 5th ed. Pacific Grove, CA: Duxbury Press; 2000.

CHAPTER 6

Ethical Considerations

LAWRENCE M. FRIEDMAN • ELEANOR B. SCHRON

This chapter will focus on selected aspects of bioethics, emphasizing ethics in the conduct of clinical trials. Extensive discussion of the many aspects of medical and research ethics and of the history of ethical standards and ethical lapses in human experimentation may be found elsewhere.[1–5] Well-known guidelines include the Nuremberg Code,[6] the Belmont Report,[7] and the World Medical Association Declaration of Helsinki.[8] In addition, there are ongoing debates, as medical science and technologic innovations outpace our understanding of and agreement on ethical issues. Much of U.S. government-supported clinical research and research conducted at institutions subject to U.S. government regulations must follow the Code of Federal Regulations, the so-called Common Rule (Title 45)[9] and/or the regulations under which the U.S. Food and Drug Administration (FDA) operates.[10] With the International Conference on Harmonisation[11] and European Union regulations,[12] there is considerable agreement internationally, but differences among countries still exist, in both law and culture. For example, the issues involving conduct of clinical research in poor or developing parts of the world have been contentious.[8,13–16]

For several reasons, clinical trials involve ethical issues beyond the usual ones in other types of clinical research. These reasons include the use of randomization, blinding (masking), the fact that many trials are international, use of interventions that are sometimes dangerous, participant consent that may not be completely informed or truly voluntary, and the need for appropriate monitoring for safety. Some of these and other selected issues will be discussed in this chapter.

BACKGROUND

Ethical considerations in clinical trials, and indeed in clinical research in general, have evolved over the past several decades. These changes occurred often in response to egregious events that, although they did not reflect the overall ethical standards of clinical research, nevertheless affected public perceptions. The Nuremberg Code[6] was developed in response to the terrible actions of doctors in Nazi Germany. It laid out standards for clinical research, the first of which is voluntary consent. Other standards included ensuring that the importance of the question being addressed justifies the risk (which should be kept to a minimum), the study is conducted by qualified investigators in appropriate facilities, the study is likely to yield meaningful results, and the subject has the right to withdraw from the study.

The World Medical Association's Declaration of Helsinki[8] was first developed in 1964, and has since been updated, most recently in 2000, with subsequent clarifications. It provides ethical principles regarding research in human subjects, including use of identifiable material and data. The ethical force of the Declaration of Helsinki is acknowledged internationally.

In the United States, several episodes of improper clinical research led to the 1974 report, Ethical Principles and Guidelines for the Protection of Human Subjects of Research (the so-called, "Belmont Report").[7] This report establishes the ethical principles of respect for persons, beneficence, and justice. These principles are applied by means of informed consent, assessment of risk and benefits, and selection of subjects.

Most clinical research in the United States is covered under parts of the Code of Federal Regulations: 45 CFR 46, the "Common Rule" that applies to much government-sponsored clinical research that is conducted at academic institutions; and 45 CFR 21, under which the Food and Drug Administration operates. An important feature of these regulations is the requirement for review of proposed clinical research by a properly constituted and functioning Institutional Review Board (IRB). In other countries such constituted groups may be known as Ethics Committees. For simplicity, in this chapter we will adopt the term used by the World Medical Association Declaration of Helsinki and the Council for International Organizations of Medical Sciences (CIOMS), ethical review committees.

Also of importance are the various International Conference on Harmonisation (ICH) guidelines.[11] These documents do not have the force of regulation, but among other aspects of drug development and testing, they establish guidance for the conduct of clinical trials in the European Union, Japan, and the United States—including ethical conduct.

INFORMED CONSENT AND ETHICAL REVIEW COMMITTEES

As noted, informed consent is a key ethical principle of the policies and regulations governing not just clinical trials, but all clinical research. A fundamental responsibility of the ethical review committee is to ensure that, except in specific circumstances or when waived for certain kinds of research, informed consent is obtained before a subject is enrolled into a study. Informed consent entails not merely providing a written consent form to be read and signed, but a process whereby the study is discussed with the subject, the subject is given an opportunity to ask questions, and sufficient time is allowed for the subject to discuss the research with family members or others before agreeing to participate. The investigator should be sure that the person being invited to participate completely understands the nature of the study and his or her obligations.

Ideally, the ethical review committee would review not just the consent form, but the full process. How often subjects truly understand the study, or even that they are in a research program, is unclear. Some have questioned the adequacy of the consent process in this regard.[17,18] The nature of the condition being studied and the kinds of subjects probably affect the extent to which the research is understood and participation is truly voluntary. For example, those in an emergency room with severe chest pain requiring morphine are not likely to be in a position to appreciate fully the advantages and disadvantages of a request to be in a clinical trial testing two approaches to reducing myocardial damage. Similarly, extra care is required for critically ill patients in intensive care units,[19] as recall of key elements may be limited.[20]

The content of the consent form may vary from country to country, and individual research institutions will have their own standards and requirements. In the United States, the basic requirements are listed in the Code of Federal Regulations[9] (Table 6.1). Among the requirements are listings of expected risks and benefits from the research and alternatives to the research. A job of the ethical review committee is to ensure that the expected risks do not outweigh the expected benefits, and that the explanations in the consent form allow subjects to make reasoned decisions on a strictly voluntary basis.

Table 6.1 Code of Federal Regulations—General Requirements for Informed Consent

Basic Elements of Informed Consent

1. A statement that the study involves research, an explanation of the purposes of the research and the expected duration of the subject's participation, a description of the procedures to be followed, and identification of any procedures which are experimental.
2. A description of any reasonably foreseeable risks or discomforts to the subject.
3. A description of any benefits to the subject or to others which may reasonably be expected from the research.
4. A disclosure of appropriate alternative procedures or courses of treatment, if any, that might be advantageous to the subject.
5. A statement describing the extent, if any, to which confidentiality of records identifying the subject will be maintained.
6. For research involving more than minimal risk, an explanation as to whether any compensation and an explanation as to whether any medical treatments are available if injury occurs and, if so, what they consist of, or where further information may be obtained.
7. An explanation of whom to contact for answers to pertinent questions about the research and research subjects' rights, and whom to contact in the event of a research-related injury to the subject.
8. A statement that participation is voluntary, refusal to participate will involve no penalty or loss of benefits to which the subject is otherwise entitled, and the subject may discontinue participation at any time without penalty or loss of benefits to which the subject is otherwise entitled.

Additional Elements of Informed Consent, When Appropriate

1. A statement that the particular treatment or procedure may involve risks to the subject (or to the embryo or fetus, if the subject is or may become pregnant) which are currently unforeseeable.
2. Anticipated circumstances under which the subject's participation may be terminated by the investigator without regard to the subject's consent.
3. Any additional costs to the subject that may result from participation in the research.
4. The consequences of a subject's decision to withdraw from the research and procedures for orderly termination of participation by the subject.
5. A statement that significant new findings developed during the course of the research which may relate to the subject's willingness to continue participation will be provided to the subject.
6. The approximate number of subjects involved in the study.

From U.S. Department of Health and Human Services. Protection of Human Subjects, Title 45 Code of Federal Regulations, Part 46. 2005.

For much research, this review process is relatively straightforward. In clinical trials, where an intervention is administered in the hopes of preventing or treating a disease or condition, one can evaluate the trade-off between the risks of the intervention and the potential benefits, along with those of any alternatives. Several situations, however, may be more problematic. One involves early-phase trials. Here, the trials are typically small and short-term, and the ability to discern clinical benefit is limited or nonexistent. The ethics of entering people into a clinical trial that holds out little or no hope of yielding benefit, but has a possibility of harm, the amount and severity of which are uncertain, has been debated.[21,22] In general, ethical review committees have approved these studies, given the need to obtain early information about potential treatments and the understanding that subjects are fully informed about the possible risks.

A second situation involves those who are incapable of giving truly informed consent. This could include children and people with intellectual or emotional limitations. With children, not only would the parents or other legal guardians need to consent and children who are able, to assent, but there are extra requirements in the United States and elsewhere; the ethical review committee may still approve the research if the risks are not greater than minimal. If the risks are greater than minimal, the study must have the prospect of direct benefit to the child and be likely to be at least as beneficial as other options or likely to lead to generalizable knowledge about the child's condition. The trial should present experiences commensurate with the child's actual or expected medical or psychosocial situations. If those situations do not apply, and the ethical review committee thinks that the research should be conducted, the Secretary of the Department of Health and Human Services must approve it.[9] Thus, with clinical trials that hold out hope of improvement or cure of a condition, the ethical review committee can decide that the balance of benefit and risks is appropriate. However, the conduct of various invasive or other potentially harmful procedures that may be important to the research, but of no obvious clinical benefit, could be precluded from the study.

For studies in others incapable of providing true consent, guidelines have been developed or proposed.[23] The ethical review committee should consider whether other safeguards, such as requiring independent monitors or others making the decisions, are needed.

A third situation involves clinical research in emergency settings. In such research, it is often impossible to obtain informed consent from the subject, or even a surrogate, until after the intervention must be initiated. The United States[24] and Canada[25] allow for emergency research as long as certain procedures are followed. These procedures include, in addition to ethical review committee approval, community consultation[26] and involvement of a data and safety monitoring committee. The situation in other parts of the world is less settled.[27]

Many clinical trials, particularly late-phase trials, are multicenter and even international. Traditionally, this has meant that the ethical review committee of each site reviews the study protocol and consent process and form. Not surprisingly, this has led to differences of opinion with regard to the specific content and wording of the consent form, and even protocol issues. Many have thought that having multiple ethical review committees reviewing the same protocol is redundant, a waste of time, and costly.[28] Others maintain that there are important reasons for ethical review committees to consider practices and cultures that might be specific to the local situation.[29] Several approaches have been advocated and attempted.[30] These range from the use of so-called central ethical review committees,[31] particularly those developed as commercial entities; to mixed models, where some sites use a central ethical review committee (especially for sites that are small or otherwise do not conduct much research) and others use local ethical review committees; to centralized review of the protocol with review at each site of the consent form and process. Most of the time, even multicenter trials that do not use a central ethical review committee employ a consent form template. That is, the study as a whole develops a model consent form that is presented to the individual ethical review committees. As long as the key elements remain, the local investigators and ethical review committees have the option to modify phrasing and make other edits appropriate to local needs.

As yet, there is no consensus as to whether central, local, or a mix is the best approach, and it is likely that institution and sponsor preferences and differences will remain, for at least some time. What is clear is that ethical review committees, whether local or central, must play an active role in ensuring that the entire consent process, indeed the entire subject accrual process, is appropriate. For example, the ethical review committee must critically review subject recruitment approaches to make sure that they are balanced and reflect accurately the goals and nature of the trial. As noted, certain circumstances, such as enrolling children and others incapable of providing true informed consent (e.g., people with intellectual or emotional limitations or in emergency research situations) require particular attention from the ethical review committee. Additionally, ethical review committees, as well as study sponsors, must be attuned to cases where there might be real or perceived undue pressure for subjects to enroll in trials. These include patients with serious conditions who are seeking any source of relief or cure. Parents of children with serious genetic abnormalities may fall into this category.

Two situations may increase these pressures. One is the so-called "therapeutic misconception."[32,33] Subjects may not fully understand that participation in a trial is a research undertaking, not a therapeutic one. Although treatment benefit may occur, that is not at all certain. The researcher's primary objective is to fulfill the requirements of the protocol, which at times may not be consistent with what the subject perceives as optimal care. A researcher who enrolls subjects who are his or her own patients may increase this therapeutic misconception. Of course, simply being a patient of a doctor who is also a researcher should not in itself disqualify someone from participating in a clinical trial. Thus extra care must be taken in this circumstance. A second situation is when the researcher has a possible conflict of interest. This could be financial (when, for example, the researcher has equity interest in the product being studied) or intellectual (when the researcher is heavily invested in a concept that has been his or her life's work). The researcher could exert undue pressures on subjects to enroll.

Ethical review committees must pay attention to these situations, just as they review the amount of payment to participants to ensure that the incentives to be in a study are appropriate. They might insist on ways to manage and reduce the likelihood of undue pressure. One way is to require that the person who approaches the prospective subject about enrollment and who explains the trial be someone other than the investigator. In some situations, a "patient advocate," someone whose primary interest is the well-being of the subject, rather than the most efficient completion of subject enrollment, might be required. These approaches can be expensive and burdensome, and can slow subject accrual. But the ethical review committee and study sponsor need to judge in what circumstances they are important.

Multicenter clinical trials, particularly international ones, entail a separate issue that ethical review committees must consider. That is, to what extent is the population served by the local site, region, or even country, likely to benefit from the information learned as a result of the trial? Are the subjects from the site being sought simply because they are convenient or likely to provide a quicker, cheaper, or clearer answer? Or are they being sought because the answer could lead to better care for the local community? This is an issue that study sponsors and investigators must address, but the ethical review committees must also consider it. They must be satisfied that the study design and goals are relevant to the population they serve. This is something that might not be fully described in the consent process. For a fuller discussion and critique of standards of conducting international trials, especially in developing countries, see Part X, Multinational Research, in *The Oxford Textbook of Clinical Research Ethics*.[5]

In addition to its role in reviewing the consent process and ensuring that the study design is both reasonable and relevant, an ethical review committee has other responsibilities. One is to make sure that the investigator team, facilities, and resources are adequate to the task of conducting the study. A study that is poorly conducted or that cannot be completed because of inadequate resources does not yield scientifically credible results. The benefits are less than planned, while the subjects are placed at the same or even greater risk.

An example of a trial that was stopped early for commercial reasons is the Controlled Onset Investigation of Cardiovascular End Points (CONVINCE), a multicenter trial comparing antihypertensive agents.[34,35] The company that sponsored the trial decided 2 years before the scheduled end that continued funding was no longer in its interest. In this situation, the investigators were committed to continued follow-up of the study participants and there is little that they or the ethical review committee could have done to foresee or prevent the company's action. However, failure to complete clinical studies for other than scientific or safety reasons is unethical.

Another responsibility is to consider the trial's data and safety monitoring plans at the time the protocol is reviewed. Even though an ethical review committee might not directly conduct such monitoring (e.g., in studies that have data and safety monitoring boards or data monitoring committees), it needs to be comfortable with the monitoring procedures that are being implemented. It should receive reports from the data and safety monitoring board after each board meeting, in order to fulfill its oversight role.

ISSUES OF CONFIDENTIALITY

Concerns over confidentiality and privacy have increased in recent years. There is no question that there are scientific, medical, and public health benefits in being able to access and merge data efficiently, quickly, and accurately. But easy access by almost anyone to individual data of all sorts, with the possibility of harm and embarrassment, has also led many to insist on protection of the data, restricting data to those viewed as having sufficient reason and proper approval.

Laws passed in the United States, Europe, and elsewhere in response to privacy concerns have been viewed by many researchers as limiting their ability to conduct clinical research.[36,37] For example, screening of patients for study eligibility, including use of databases from specialized units or laboratories and chart review, has been questioned or made more onerous. Follow-up of study subjects after the actual study has ended might be useful, or even important for patient health. Yet unless clearly allowed in the consent form, such follow-up might not be possible. Study subjects may drop out of the trial and may decide to rescind their agreement to participate. In such cases, "passive" follow-up, something that at one time was quite readily accomplished by access to hospital records or other databases, may now be forbidden by policies and regulations.

Genetic data are now obtained in many clinical trials, and tissue or serum specimens are collected and archived. These practices have implications for future, unspecified uses of the data and material, some of which might be contrary to the expressed consent and wishes of the participants. More difficult is the fact that genetic information on a study subject will convey information about families or even communities. American Indian tribes, for example, have been quite vocal about their rights as communities, beyond the rights of the individual members of the tribes.[38] Even if the information is made anonymous, there are fears that privacy and confidentiality cannot be ensured. With enhanced availability of data about individuals in all sorts of electronic formats, even if clinical research studies delete obvious individual identifiers, complete privacy may not be possible. Inappropriate access and use of these data by researchers, health insurers, or government bodies is a major concern.

Some of the issues identified above reflect the newness of the policies and regulations, and the natural concerns of many that information can and will be abused. Ethical review committees have taken very different stances and approaches to these policies. These differences will likely attenuate as more experience is gained with the policies. In the United States both the Federal Government and many states have passed laws to prevent the use of genetic data for discrimination by insurers or employers.[39] Certificates of Confidentiality may allow investigators to refuse to yield data on subjects, although these may be limited in scope and effect.[40]

Privacy concerns are magnified by several important activities. The U.S. National Institutes of Health now encourage, and in some cases mandate, sharing of data and specimens from studies that they fund.[41]

Because the studies are conducted with public funds, researchers other than the original investigators should have the right to access and use data and specimens, once the original investigators have been given a reasonable time to report their findings.[42] Specimens and databanks have been and are being developed by various groups, with the intent of allowing public (or at least responsible investigator) use. If these resources are to be maximally useful, there must be ways of merging, for example, phenotypic and genotypic data. Even though name, address, Social Security numbers, and other identifiers are removed, there may still be ways for the recipient to learn the identity of the individual.

Many large clinical trials are international. Regulations and databases, and therefore the ability to identify and follow study participants, will differ among nations. Short of having a study policy of adhering to the procedures of the most restrictive country, there will be inconsistencies in things such as completeness of follow-up, long-term assessment, and use of genetic data. Study investigators will need to recognize and develop approaches to handling these differences at the beginning of the study.

There are no perfect solutions to these problems. Researchers and study participants will both need to understand the limitations of privacy and confidentiality protections, and act within the scope of what is feasible. That means that consent must be as complete and understandable as possible, with the ability to "opt out"; that researchers and staff must undergo rigorous training in research ethics and the imperatives of maintaining subject privacy, respect, and autonomy; that ethical review committees and study sponsors must appropriately consider both the needs of the study and the rights of participants; and that we think long-term, to what may occur beyond the termination of the trial itself.

TRIAL FUTILITY

There is an extensive literature on the rationale for and approaches to data and safety monitoring in clinical trials. In essence, ethical imperatives require that whenever we conduct clinical research, we not only design the studies to minimize risks to participants but we regularly assess the conduct of the studies to ensure that indeed the risks are not greater than projected or greater than the anticipated benefits. In clinical trials, where possibly harmful interventions are being administered, this imperative is even greater than in several other sorts of clinical research. A common approach is to have an individual or group monitor the ongoing progress of the trial and the accumulating data. Those interested in further details and case studies are referred to other sources.[43,44]

Here, one issue relevant to data and safety monitoring will be discussed. When the investigator designs a trial, he or she makes assumptions about event rate or mean change in the control group, hoped for or expected effect of the intervention, level of lack of compliance to the protocol among those in the control and intervention groups, amount of missing data, and any other factor that affects sample size. In addition, the investigator decides on appropriate Type 1 (α) and Type 2 (β) errors, β being 1 $-$ power. The assumptions made may be based on data from earlier small trials, observational studies, what is thought to be a clinically meaningful result, or simply what is feasible given the available time and resources. Inevitably, one or more of the assumptions will turn out to be incorrect; unfortunately, typically in the direction of making it less likely that a clear study outcome will be found. If these estimates are so far off from what is observed once the study gets underway that it is unlikely that the study will come to a clear answer, judgment must be made as to the purpose of continuing the study. After all, putting participants at risk with little hope of learning something important is a violation of ethical standards and is inconsistent with what was communicated to the participants when they enrolled.

As always, however, making this judgment is not simple, and may involve several approaches. One approach is to consider what has been termed, "unconditional power."[45] If, for example, enrollment of subjects is slower than planned, using the original event and effect estimates one can calculate how much lower the power will be. Rather than 80% or 90%, with the original sample size, it may be 70% or even much lower. Of course, other factors may not be as originally estimated. The control group event rate and/or the treatment effect may be greater than expected. Similarly, compliance to the study protocol may be better. Therefore, the lower number of participants may be adequate to answer the question. Calculations based on observed data have been termed "conditional power." Here, what has occurred in the trial up until the time of the analysis is considered. One can calculate whether, given reasonable assumptions as to future data, the study is worth continuing. If future data are very unlikely to alter study conclusions, then it may be reasonable to stop the trial. If the study experience up to now, taking into account unconditional and conditional power, is such that there is a very low probability of coming up with an answer, or of declaring a new treatment to be better than control, it may be futile to continue. Given the expense and effort on the part of the investigators—and most important, the risks and possible burdens to which study participants are being put—the study should be stopped.

An example is the Cooperative New Scandinavian Enalapril Survival Study II (CONSENSUS II).[46,47] This study looked at whether enalapril given at the time of an acute myocardial infarction would reduce mortality. The trial's Data and Safety Monitoring Committee decided at the beginning that the study should be ended if accumulating data indicated that the final result was unlikely to show significant benefit from enalapril. The monitoring committee noted a nonsignificant trend against enalapril early in the trial. This trend persisted, and even though the predetermined futility boundary had not been crossed, the low likelihood of seeing benefit and safety concerns led the committee to recommend trial termination.

Of course, such decisions are rarely straightforward. Usually, although there is a primary trial endpoint, there are other outcomes of interest and importance. The power to answer the primary endpoint may be much lower than expected, but other outcomes may still be feasibly answered. Whether the importance of these other outcomes outweighs the potential harms must be evaluated. Also important is what was understood by the participants during the consent process. They may have signed on to a trial looking at mortality from heart disease, but may not have agreed to a trial looking at angina pectoris as an outcome. The data and safety monitoring board must assess all of these factors when making its recommendation to continue, modify, or end a trial, keeping in mind that its primary responsibility is to the study subjects.

SUMMARY

Ethical considerations in clinical trials, indeed in clinical research in general, involve many aspects, only a few of which are addressed in this chapter. In addition, ethical standards are evolving and laws are changing to meet scientific and technical advances and cultural needs. Nevertheless, key factors remain. They include the need for full and open voluntary consent, the need to consider both participant interests and those of society, the need for ongoing education of the entire investigator team, and a process for oversight and adjudication, when the inevitable conflicts between interests arise.

REFERENCES

1. Levine RJ. *Ethics and Regulation of Clinical Research*. 2nd ed. New Haven: Yale University Press; 1988.
2. Brody BA. *The Ethics of Biomedical Research: An International Perspective*. New York: Oxford University Press; 1998.
3. Emanuel EJ, Crouch RA, Arras JD, et al., eds. *Ethical and Regulatory Aspects of Clinical Research: Readings and Commentary*. Baltimore: Johns Hopkins University Press; 2003.
4. Piantadosi S. Ethical Considerations. *Clinical Trials: A Methodologic Perspective*. New York: Wiley; 1997:29–60.
5. Emanuel EJ, Grady C, Crouch RA, et al. *The Oxford Textbook of Clinical Research Ethics*. New York: Oxford University Press; 2008.
6. Nuremberg Code. *Trials of War Criminals Before the Nuremberg Military Tribunals under Control Council Law No. 10*. Vol. 2. Washington, DC: U.S. Government Printing Office; 1949:181–182.
7. The National Commission for the Protection of Human Subjects of Biomedical and Behavioral Research. *The Belmont Report: Ethical Principles and Guidelines for the Protection of Human Subjects of Research*. http://www.hhs.gov/ohrp/humansubjects/guidance/belmont.htm. 1979.
8. World Medical Association. *Declaration of Helsinki*. http://www.wma.net/e/policy/b3.htm. 2000.
9. U.S. Department of Health and Human Services. Protection of Human Subjects, Title 45 Code of Federal Regulations, Part 46. http://www.hhs.gov/ohrp/humansubjects/guidance/45cfr46.htm#subparta. 2005.
10. U.S. Food and Drug Administration. Federal Food, Drug, and Cosmetic Act. http://www.fda.gov/opacom/laws/fdcact/fdctoc.htm. 2004.
11. The ICH Steering Committee. International Conference on Harmonisation. http://www.ich.org/cache/compo/276-254-1.html. 2007.
12. European Medicines Agency. Scientific Guidelines for Human Medicinal Products. http://www.emea.europa.eu/htms/human/humanguidelines/efficacy.htm. 2007.
13. Lurie P, Wolfe SM. Unethical trials of interventions to reduce perinatal transmission of the human immunodeficiency virus in developing countries. *N Engl J Med*. 1997;337:853–856.
14. Annas GJ, Grodin MA. Human rights and maternal-fetal HIV transmission prevention trials in Africa. *Am J Public Health*. 1998;88:560–563.
15. Crouch RA, Arras JD. AZT trials and tribulations. *Hastings Cent Rep*. 1998;28:26–34.
16. Killen J. Ethics of clinical research in the developing world. *Nat Rev Immunol*. 2002;2:210.
17. Davis TC, Holcombe RF, Berkel HJ, et al. Informed consent for clinical trials: a comparative study of standard versus simplified forms. *J Natl Cancer Inst*. 1998;90:668–674.

18. Joffe S, Cook EF, Cleary PD, et al. Quality of informed consent: a new measure of understanding among research subjects. *J Natl Cancer Inst.* 2001; 93:139–147.
19. American Thoracic Society. The ethical conduct of clinical research involving critically ill patients in the United States and Canada: principles and recommendations. *Am J Respir Crit Care Med.* 2004;170:1375–1384.
20. Chenaud C, Merlani P, Luyasu S, et al. Informed consent for research obtained during the intensive care unit stay. *Crit Care.* 2006;10(6)R170.
21. Agrawal M, Emanuel EJ. Ethics of phase 1 oncology studies: reexamining the arguments and data. *JAMA.* 2003;290:1075–1082.
22. Joffe S, Miller FG. Rethinking risk-benefit assessment for phase I cancer trials. *J Clin Oncol.* 2006;24:2987–2990.
23. Wendler D. Core safeguards for clinical research with adults who are unable to consent. *Ann Intern Med.* 2001;135:514–523.
24. U.S. Food and Drug Administration. Exception from informed consent requirements for emergency research; Title 21 CFR Part 50. http://www.accessdata.fda.gov/scripts/cdrh/cfdocs/cfcfr/CFRSearch.cfm?fr=50.24. 2006.
25. Government of Canada. Interagency Advisory Panel on Research Ethics. Tri-Council Policy Statement (TCPS): Ethical Conduct for Research Involving Humans. http://www.pre.ethics.gc.ca/english/policystatement/section2.cfm#2F. 2001.
26. Richardson LD, Quest TE, Birnbaum S. Communicating with communities about emergency research. *Acad Emerg Med.* 2005;12:1064–1070.
27. Coats TJ, Shakur H. Consent in emergency research: new regulations. *Emerg Med J.* 2005;22:683–685.
28. Burman WJ. Breaking the camel's back: multicenter clinical trials and local institutional review boards. *Ann Intern Med.* 2001;134:152–157.
29. Levine RJ. Institutional review boards: a crisis in confidence. *Ann Intern Med.* 2001;134:161–163.
30. National Conference on Alternative IRB Models. Optimizing Human Subject Protection. Washington, DC. 2006.
31. Christian MC, Goldberg JL, Killen J, et al. A central institutional review board for multi-institutional trials. *N Engl J Med.* 2002;346:1405–1408.
32. Henderson GE, Easter MM, Zimmer C, et al. Therapeutic misconception in early phase gene transfer trials. *Soc Sci Med.* 2006;62:239–253.
33. Appelbaum PS, Roth LH, Lidz C. The therapeutic misconception: informed consent in psychiatric research. *Int J Law Psychiatry.* 1982;5:319–329.
34. Psaty BM, Rennie D. Stopping medical research to save money: a broken pact with researchers and patients. *JAMA.* 2003;289:2128–2131.
35. Black HR, Elliott WJ, Grandits G, et al. Principal results of the Controlled Onset Verapamil Investigation of Cardiovascular End Points (CONVINCE) trial. *JAMA.* 2003;289:2073–2082.
36. National Institutes of Health. Clinical Research and the HIPAA Privacy Rule. http://privacyruleandresearch.nih.gov/clin_research.rtf . 2003.

37. Trevena L, Irwig L, Barratt A. Impact of privacy legislation on the number and characteristics of people who are recruited for research: a randomized controlled trial. *J Med Ethics*. 2006;32:473–477.
38. Foster MW, Bernsten D, Carter TH. A model agreement for genetic research in socially identifiable populations. *Am J Hum Genet*. 1998;63:696–702.
39. Human Genome Project Information: Genetics Privacy and Legislation. hhtp://www.ornl.gov/sci/techresources/Human_Genome/elsi/legislat.shtml. 2008
40. NIH Office of Extramural Research. Certificates of Confidentiality Kiosk. http://grants.nih.gov/grants/policy/coc/faqs.htm. 2006.
41. NIH Office of Extramural Research. NIH Data Sharing Policy. http://grants.nih.gov/grants/policy/data_sharing/. 2007.
42. Geller NL, Sorlie P, Coady S, et al. Limited access data sets from studies funded by the National Heart, Lung, and Blood Institute. *Clin Trials*. 2004;1:517–524.
43. DeMets DL, Furberg C, Friedman LM. *Data Monitoring in Clinical Trials: A Case Studies Approach*. New York: Springer; 2006.
44. Ellenberg SS, Fleming TR, DeMets DL. *Data Monitoring Committees in Clinical Trials: A Practical Perspective*. West Sussex: Wiley; 2003.
45. Proschan MA, Lan KKG, Wittes JT. *Statistical Monitoring of Clinical Trials: A Unified Approach*. New York: Springer; 2006.
46. Swedberg K. Effects of the early administration of enalapril on mortality in patients with acute myocardial infarction. Results of the Cooperative New Scandinavian Enalapril Survival Study II (CONSENSUS II). *N Engl J Med*. 1992;327:678–684.
47. Snapinn S, Furberg CD. Stopping a trial for futility: the Cooperative New Scandinavian Enalapril Survival Study II. In: DeMets DL, Furberg CD, Friedman LM, eds. *Data Monitoring in Clinical Trials: A Case Studies Approach*. New York: Springer; 2006:302–311.

SECTION II

Large Multicenter Trials: Structure and Conduct

CHAPTER 7

Study Organization and Governance

FLEUR HUDSON • JULIE BAKOBAKI • ABDEL BABIKER

There are a number of reasons why we might want to conduct a multisite clinical trial: it is often not possible to recruit sufficient numbers of volunteers from one center to reliably answer the question addressed by the trial; it may not be logistically possible to recruit all volunteers from one center; we may want to include volunteers from different regions or countries to ensure that the results are widely generalizable; or there may be a wish to further scientific collaborations by including multiple groups in the planning and execution of the trial.

The more centers that are involved in a trial, the less straightforward its planning becomes. International trials have added layers of complexity as national regulatory requirements, trial governance, and logistical organization need to be taken into account. Additional financial resources, drug delivery, and data management logistics required to run such a trial need careful consideration.

There are advantages in terms of increased relevance of results that occur from conducting the trial in an ethnically and geographically diverse population. Different regulatory procedures in different countries increase the time required for trial setup. Where an international trial is intended, such issues escalate. Even within the European Community, different member countries vary in their interpretation of the European Union (EU) clinical trials directive and subsequent regulatory requirements governing the conduct of studies. Understanding of the different regulations and an agreed equivalence between corresponding national regulatory bodies is desirable for the successful completion of a trial.

All clinical trials must be conducted according to the Principles of Good Clinical Practice (GCP).[1] This is a set of guidelines developed to provide a unified standard across the European Union, Japan, and the

United States, which was labeled ICH GCP at the International Conference on Harmonisation in 1996. GCP forms an international ethical and scientific quality standard for the design, conduct, performance, monitoring, audit, recording, analysis, and reporting of clinical trials that involve human participants, to ensure the protection of the safety, rights, and confidentiality of trial participants, and to maintain the integrity, credibility, and accuracy of clinical trial data.

Although other regulatory bodies in other countries outside of the European Union, Japan, and the United States also follow ICH GCP principles—either using the guidelines as they are written or, as with the Medicines Control Council in South Africa, publishing their own guidelines interpreting them.[2] It is essential that each country's GCP guidance is followed as appropriate; it is a good idea to assess where any country-specific differences lie in the planning phase so that a justification for the procedures to be followed in the trial can be prepared and local regulatory bodies advised accordingly. It may be that the trial procedures differ from country to country in order to meet local requirements. With careful assessment and preparation this need not have any impact on the results of the trial.

However a clinical trial is organized, trial governance, GCP, and successful coordination of all the regulatory requirements is of paramount importance. This chapter highlights the considerations to be made and the systems needed for the successful running of a multisite clinical trial in today's regulatory environment.

MULTISITE TRIAL ORGANIZATION

In order to comply with GCP a trial sponsor will ensure that all the numerous regulatory and ethical approvals required are obtained and that trial governance procedures are in place for the entire duration of the trial.

Regulatory Agencies and Clinical Trial Authorizations

Before a clinical trial can commence there are a number of approvals that have to be obtained. Regulatory agencies are country or region-wide (within a country) independent bodies that operate in a variety of ways issuing guidance (and in some cases requirements and with enforcement abilities) on medicines and medical devices. They aim to ensure that new medicines or devices are only allowed onto the market with a license or marketing authorization *if there is enough evidence that the potential benefits will outweigh the likely risks to patients*. They also ensure that the product's safety and efficacy or performance has been assessed. This assessment takes place through the collection and analysis of clinical trial data. Regulatory agencies aim to ensure that acceptable levels of protection are provided to trial participants through appropriate trial design and conduct.

Regulatory agencies define how the public is able to access products, dependent upon the level of risk the product poses if inappropriately used. For example, medicines can be made available for purchase without a prescription, under the supervision of a pharmacist, or with a prescription from a health care provider. These agencies ensure that information provided with an approved medicine or device is appropriate for the user, readable, and fits the safety and efficacy profile based on the available supporting data.

Regulatory agencies receive information from health care professionals, pharmaceutical companies, patients, and the public about adverse events from medicines and devices that are in use. This ongoing data collection allows an assessment of their continued appropriateness, safety, and efficacy. It also allows a review of the product's manufacturing or supply quality, and enables the restriction or withdrawal of products from use. Advice or warnings are issued by regulatory agencies if new or updated information about an adverse effect, manufacturer, supply, or instructions for use of a product needs communicating to health care professionals or the public.

Because of the large amount of up-to-date safety and efficacy information that they collect, regulatory agencies are able to give advice to professionals and the public about the appropriateness of use of medicines and devices, and particularly about the adequacy of their maintenance, sterility, or testing.

Other roles that regulatory agencies play are in prevention or disruption of the supply of unauthorized or counterfeit medicines and devices; discouragement of inappropriate sales of second-hand devices; inspection of the coordinating centers and investigational sites conducting required clinical trials; and making appropriate information available to the public.

In most countries, regulatory approvals—Clinical Trial Authorizations (CTAs)—are required when a clinical trial uses an Investigational Medicinal Product (IMP), in the United States an Investigational Device Exemption (IDE), or an Investigational New Drug (IND). An IMP/IND is one where there is no existing license for use of the product/drug; where it has a license but it is being tested for a new indication (e.g., a cancer drug that is currently licensed for use in treating patients with lung cancer, but not in other cancers is being considered for additional cancers); where there is a change in the approved route of administration or dosage level; or where there is a change in the approved patient population (e.g., children or a population at greater risk such as the elderly, HIV-positive patients, or the immunocompromised). CTA/IND applications are made to the relevant regulatory body by the individual or group who will act as the sponsor for the trial. As CTAs/INDs are region or country specific, international collaborations may involve more than one CTA/IND per trial. The CTA/IND is held by the group taking sponsor responsibilities for the trial in a particular country or region. It must abide by the regulations set out by each of the regulatory authorities that grant the authorizations.

There are a number of websites available with information on the requirements for regulatory approvals. In the United Kingdom, the MHRA has an easily accessible algorithm that can be found on http://www.ec.europa.eu; outside of the United Kingdom in the European Union, all of the information required by each member state's competent authority (regulatory body) can be found on http://www.eudract.emea.europa.eu; and a list of regulatory authorities websites for countries outside of the European Union can be found on http://www.pharmweb.net/pwmirror/pwk/pharmwebk.html. In the United States, the Food and Drug Administration (FDA) regulations and guidelines can be found on http://www.fda.gov. In Canada, Health Canada regulations are located at http://www.hc-sc.gc.ca.

Ethics Committees and Institutional Review Boards

When undertaking clinical research it is essential that trial participants be treated fairly, humanely, and without being placed in any unnecessary danger. In order to judge the ethical implications of research it must be approved by an independent committee.

The need for ethical assessment of clinical research was borne out of poor research practices having serious outcomes for participants. The Tuskegee Syphilis Study[3,4] carried out in the United States involved syphilis patients being denied treatment for their condition—something that would not be allowed today. The widespread use of thalidomide as a treatment for morning sickness in pregnant women led to many seriously disabled children being born in the 1960s.[5,6] Modern research is thus strictly regulated to ensure the protection of the rights, safety, dignity, and well-being of human subjects participating in clinical trials.

Before initiating a trial, ethics approval must be gained from the relevant authority in the country where the research will be conducted. This authority or committee will review the proposed project plan, the trial protocol, and other documents to assess the design, relevance, and applicability to practice. The proposed research will be assessed to ensure that it complies with all applicable laws within the area represented by the committee, and that it does not breach standards of professional conduct and practice.

The organization of Ethics Committees (ECs) and Institutional Review Boards (IRBs) varies widely across the world, but they may be independent, governmental, or commercial. Generally, larger, national organizational bodies maintain standards by guidance and management support to smaller committees, preparing frameworks and quality assurance for research assessment. While specific committees review specific trials, the larger framework in which they operate will promote the design of ethical research more widely.

It is desirable that ECs/IRBs be made up of people from a wide range of cultures and communities, as well as being representative of gender and race. For specific studies researching a particular population, it is important that the committee includes a member representative of, or someone who has experience working with, that community (e.g., prisoners or the mentally impaired). These committees are notable for their diversity of membership, which allows for the research to be assessed from a wide range of perspectives. Along with health care professionals—nurses, clinicians, and pharmacists—there are patients, members of the public, and academics. Members should be specially trained in research ethics and should be independent of the researcher, funder, or host of any research project under review. Often outside expertise may be brought in for advice, but these advisers will not take part in any voting.

Applications to these committees are specific to the country of research. However, an application will generally comprise of a comprehensive application form that should be sent in with the protocol and other supporting documentation.

Once the application is made, it will be reviewed and a response provided in writing. The assessment of the committee will be one of the following: approval, modifications required prior to approval, or disapproval. For trial amendments, the committee may also respond with a termination or suspension of any prior approval.

Profiles of new drugs are assessed to ensure that relevant safeguards are in place. The suitability of the principle investigator will also be assessed by reviewing his or her qualifications and background. Once the trial is running, the committee ensures the ongoing welfare of patients by reviewing regular reports. Any amendments to the trial protocol or supporting documents require further assessment and approval by the committee before they can be implemented. The exception to this is when the amendment must be implemented immediately for patient safety (e.g., as a result of a recommendation from the trial's Data Monitoring Committee).

Although ensuring the ongoing safety of the participants once enrolled in the research is part of the committee's mandate, the committee is not privy to data on treatment differences in safety parameters during follow-up. There are ongoing discussions about whether these committees should be reviewing ongoing listings of some or all adverse events, or whether such information should only be reviewed by Data Monitoring Committees (discussed further below).

TRIAL GOVERNANCE

Trial governance is the term used for the collective oversight bodies formed for each clinical trial. Although the ultimate oversight responsibility rests with the sponsor, for practical reasons the sponsor's responsibilities are usually delegated to various groups and individuals. Depending on the extent of the sponsor's direct involvement with delegation of responsibilities, a number of committees are involved in trial governance: the Trial Steering Committee (TSC, SC) or Executive Committee (ExC, EC); the Data Monitoring Committee (DMC); and the Trial Management Group (TMG) or the protocol team (PT)—sometimes given different titles (Fig. 7.1). They ensure that the trial is being conducted in accordance with the protocol and procedures approved by the ethics committee and regulatory authorities, and offer independent guidance on trial management. Specialized trial subcommittees may also be convened to advise on specific substudies or areas of work. For example, there might be a translational research, quality-of-life, or health economics subgroup whose committee will advise on these aspects of trial management and comment on proposals for further research into these areas.

It has been found helpful for each of these committees/groups to have its own charter—a written document, signed off by the group members, to describe the membership, terms of reference, roles, responsibilities, authority, decision-making, and relationships to other relevant groups involved in the trial's oversight. The charter defines the format, timing, and frequency of meetings. It also includes details of the group's responsibilities at different time-points throughout the lifetime of the trial and the method and frequency of trial documentation required for reporting to the group. Central to the functioning of these oversight bodies is the

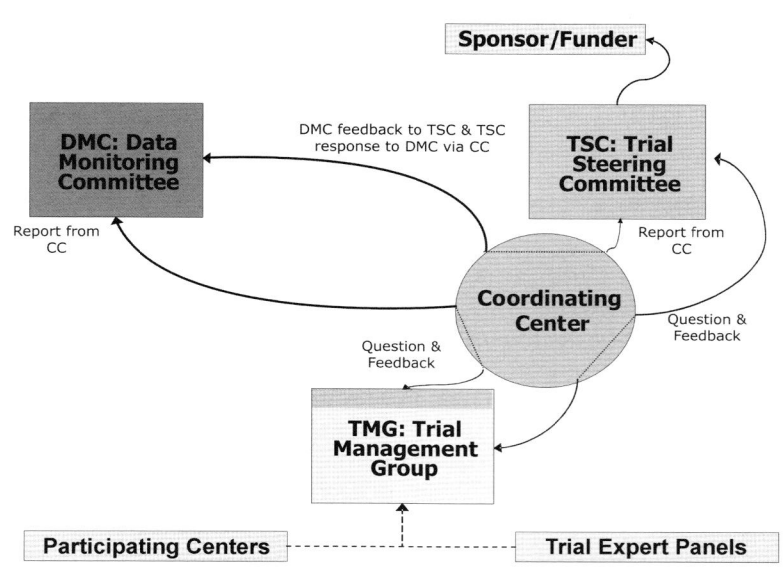

FIGURE 7.1 Diagram of how all the groups fit together and feed into each other.

study coordinating center, typically responsible for clinical sites coordination, data management, and statistical analyses.

Trial Oversight: Steering Committee (TSC, SC)/ Executive Committee (ExC, EC)

This overarching committee is appointed by (and acts on behalf of) the sponsor to provide oversight of the progress of the trial and to ensure it is conducted in accordance with the principles of GCP. In addition to providing expert oversight of the study, this committee's specific roles include approval of the trial protocol and any subsequent amendments before submission to the appropriate ethics committees, reviewing regular reports of the study progress from the TMG, assessing the relevance and impact of any accumulating external evidence, and making decisions as to the future continuation of the trial usually after recommendation from the independent DMC. It has a central role in communicating with the sponsor/funder, the TMG, the DMC, and the investigators conducting the trial.

Membership of the trial oversight committee usually includes the leadership of the TMG (e.g., the principal investigator(s), a senior trial statistician, and the trial physician or medical officer). Some sponsors recommend that this committee has an independent chair plus at least two other independent members. Geographical/national representation in the membership is highly recommended, particularly in international trials. It is frequently recommended that this committee have at least one member from a relevant consumer group, who will represent the participant groups likely to be affected by the trial.

Independent Data (and Safety) Monitoring Committee (DMC or DSMC)

The ethical and scientific need for monitoring accumulating data has been recognized since the early days of development of the modern randomized trial more than four decades ago. However, it was acknowledged that knowledge of trends in accumulating data by the investigators could undermine their relationship with other participating clinicians, jeopardize their ability to recruit their own patients, and negatively affect the integrity of the study. In addition, repeated comparative statistical tests require some adjustment so as not to increase the rate of false-positive conclusions (Type 1 error) of a treatment effect when none exists. This has led to the establishment of independent data monitoring committees and the development of appropriate statistical methods for monitoring clinical trials. The organization, roles, responsibilities, and operating procedures of the DMC are briefly discussed below.

A DMC is a group of independent experts that examines various aspects of the accumulated data at different stages of the trial, and reports to the oversight committee and/or sponsor on the appropriateness or otherwise of continuation of the study. The purpose of a DMC is to ensure the continuing safety of trial participants and to protect the integrity of the trial results. This safeguard not only protects those participants enrolled in the trial but also the population of patients that the trial findings will affect. The DMC functions by periodically monitoring the main outcome measures (safety and efficacy) and the overall conduct of the trial (data validity). This is the committee that is in the best position to recommend the immediate termination of a trial.

Although there is no standard format suitable for all trials, there are generally accepted guidelines for DMC operations.[7,9,10,13,14,16]

Which Trials Need a DMC?

Although all trials require monitoring, the establishment of an independent DMC is not necessary for all trials. In 1998, the U.S. National Institutes of Health (NIH) issued a policy that all multicenter phase III trials must have an independent, external DMC. Although a DMC is now widely used in trials of all phases, in the case of relatively small or low-risk studies the TSC may also assume the role of the DMC.

DMC Responsibilities

The main responsibilities of the DMC are to safeguard the interests of trial participants, assess safety and efficacy of the interventions during the trial, and monitor the overall conduct of the study.

DMC Composition

The DMC should have multidisciplinary representation. This will involve at least one clinician with expertise in the disease area of the study and at least one statistician. Some DMCs include lay members with experience in heath education, law, medical ethics, and so forth. Although some national/regional representation in the membership of DMCs for multinational trials would be desirable, this is not as important as for the membership of the oversight committee. Experience and expertise should be the guiding principle for the choice of DMC members, and it is strongly recommended that at least the chairperson and one statistician have experience in clinical trials and DMC operations. The size of DMCs varies considerably in reported trials—some with as few as 3 members and others with as many as 20.[7] The DAMOCLES Group recommends a DMC membership between 4 and 6 with additional members coopted to meetings as necessary.[6] DMC members should be free of any financial or professional conflict of interest.

Specific Role: To Stop or Not to Stop the Trial

The DMC should undertake interim review of study progress, including recruitment; data quality; adherence to the protocol; and primary, secondary, and safety outcome data. On the basis of this review, the DMC makes recommendations to the oversight committee and/or sponsor about continuing, terminating, or modifying the trial. The committee may recommend early termination for all or some patients if the interim results provide clear evidence of significant clinical benefit or harm. The trial may also be terminated early if interim data indicate a low probability of achieving the trial objectives. The decision to recommend termination of the study is complex and should not be based solely on the statistical criteria used for formal interim analyses. Other considerations include external evidence that obviates the need for the trial; outcome rates so different from those expected that the trial is either not feasible or not needed; and inability to enroll required numbers in a practicable time-frame.

The DMC Charter

It is desirable that each DMC have a document outlining its roles, responsibilities, and operational procedure. This document should include details of membership; frequency and format of meetings; and specific roles of the committee. It should also detail the statistical monitoring guidelines including the frequency and timing of interim analyses and provide a summary of the contents of the interim reports. The charter must be ratified by both the oversight committee and/or sponsor as well as the DMC at its first meeting, preferably before the start of the trial. Detailed suggestions for the contents of a DMC charter can be found in publications by the DAMOCLES Study Group.[6,8,10]

The Regulatory Imperative

The International Conference on Harmonisation Efficacy topic 9 (ICH E9) recommends an independent DMC (with written operating procedures and recorded minutes of meetings) for many clinical trials. The FDA draft guidance (2002) states that an independent DMC enhances the credibility of the trial's findings and "protects the sponsor (and thus the trial) from pressure towards premature disclosure of results due to the Securities and Exchange Commission (SEC) requirements, fiduciary responsibility or other business considerations" (FDA draft guidance (2002).[9]

Monitoring procedures as part of the protocol are reviewed by the FDA for all trials of drugs that are not licensed in the dosage or for the indications used in the trial. The EU Directive requires protocol review by regulatory bodies in Europe. Both ICH E9 and the FDA draft guidance document state that all DMC meeting records should be submitted to the regulatory body. However, regulatory bodies do not typically have access to interim data unless the data are known by the sponsor at the time of the interim analysis. Formal interim analyses require direct comparison of trial outcomes. This involves very sensitive information that should have very restricted distribution—essentially the DMC and the trial or independent statistician responsible for analyses in the report.

TRIAL MANAGEMENT GROUP (TMG)/ PROTOCOL TEAM (PT)

The Trial Management Group (also sometimes called the Protocol Team) is responsible for leading all activities associated with trial management. Its responsibilities include providing clinical and other expert guidance to the coordinating center and participating sites in protocol- related matters;

developing strategies to facilitate timely enrollment, retention, and adherence to the protocol; and reporting to the TSC and DMC on the conduct of the study. The TMG is led by the principal investigator or the protocol chair. To ensure that the multiple departments involved in trial management are represented, members include the principal (and co-principal) investigator(s), project leader, trial statistician(s), trial coordinator, and other investigators providing relevant specific expertise (e.g., pharmacy and laboratory issues).

The group should meet frequently at the beginning of the trial and thereafter meet at least quarterly.

In trial networks, with more than one trial implemented at a number of sites, this committee is replicated for each protocol and led by the protocol chair. For single trials this committee may be subsumed by the Steering Committee or Executive Committee.

THE TRIAL COORDINATING CENTER: FUNCTION AND ORGANIZATION

The trial Coordinating Center (CC) is responsible for the day-to-day management of the trial-protocol management, sites coordination, data management (including development of case report forms [CRFs] and setting up and maintaining the trial database), and statistical analyses, and provides regular reports to the TMG(s), TSC, and DMC. A single coordinating center responsible for protocol implementation—ensuring that all regulatory requirements are met and dealing directly with clinical sites for receipt of case report forms and resolution of data queries—is efficient and works well for a trial conducted in one country. It is sometimes adopted in multinational trials, particularly in studies conducted by pharmaceutical companies for drug registration. There are several major disadvantages of this model that can have significant impact on enrollment, retention, and data quality if applied to collaborative international trials. It provides no sense of ownership of the study by the participating collaborating country-specific groups, which in turn leads to lack of motivation from these groups to exert sufficient effort in the conduct of the study. Differences in language, culture, regulatory procedures, and the way health care systems operate in different countries require customized procedures for trial implementation that are best dealt with nationally.

Other models for trial coordination that address the issue of ownership and enhance the collaborative spirit among the investigators to a varying degree have been adopted by several trial networks. The common theme is the establishment of regional and/or national coordinating centers responsible for the conduct of the trial in their region/country with one of these centers acting as an Overall Coordinating Center (OCC) for the trial. This allows local problems to be identified quickly, helps instill a sense of ownership in the collaborating centers, and has obvious advantages in terms of local capacity strengthening in situations where some of the participating countries lack extensive experience in the conduct of clinical trials. A notable variation between the networks which have adopted such a global structure for study coordination is the extent to which data management is centralized. The following are examples of study coordination models adopted by some trial networks:

1. Figure 7.2 gives a schematic description for the structure used by the International Network for Strategic Initiatives in Global HIV Trials (INSIGHT) in trial coordination. The coordination of over 300 clinical sites in INSIGHT is achieved through a lead OCC in Minneapolis working closely with four international coordinating centers (ICCs) in Copenhagen, London, Sydney, and Washington. Each ICC is responsible for study coordination in several countries through several site/national coordinating centers. A single database is set up at the overall coordinating center, and case report forms (CRFs) are transmitted from the clinical sites to the overall coordinating center via the regional/national CCs.

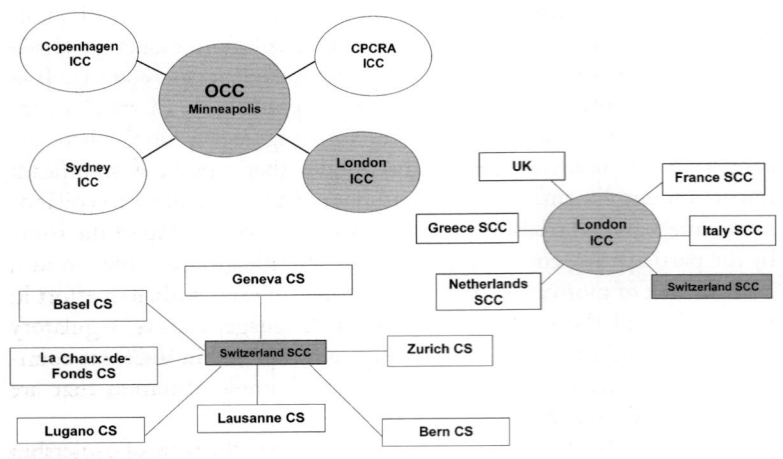

FIGURE 7.2 Trial coordination in the INSIGHT network.

2. The DART trial[17] has an overall coordinating center in London working with three national coordinating centers in Uganda and Zimbabwe. Using a common database management system, each national CC uploads all tables to a central database at the OCC frequently. The clinical database for the DART trial was a custom-made solution to some of the constraints and opportunities presented by doing a large-scale study in three major centers in Africa, with data coordination and primary analysis at the OCC in London, starting in 2003.

These factors included:

- A desire to build capacity and empower national coordinating centers.
- Large amounts of data entry required, in as real time as possible.
- Uncertain Internet connections at sites.
- Uncertain IT and database experience at sites.
- Requirements of data protection and QA.

The chosen solution was to use an SQL Server 2000 database, which provided appropriate security and was affordable, scalable, and reasonably easy to install and maintain. For data entry, an MS Access application was developed, which had the advantage of familiarity to users of other MS Office products. An SQL Server was installed at each center in Africa and at the CTU in London, and data are transferred to London twice every 2 weeks mostly by file transfer protocol (ftp) transfer.

In London the individual site databases are recreated, validated, and merged into a single database with validation checks. This database also has some data records entered at OCC (e.g., end point review data). Analysis files are generated from this merged dataset, which is also used for regular data checks to identify data problems, as well as for interim and final analyses.

3. In the Initio trial,[18,19] multiple experienced regional/national coordinating centers in London (OCC), Paris, Rome, Marburg, and Sydney were used. These centers had even more autonomy than the coordinating centers in the DART trial and the INSIGHT network, each taking on some sponsor responsibilities for the conduct of the study in their region/country. The randomization schedule was generated by the OCC in London, and common CRFs were used by all sites. However, each regional/national CC was responsible for the management of data from its site, and a prespecified set of analysis files was transmitted periodically (every 3 months) to the OCC in London.

> **ROLE OF TRIAL COORDINATING CENTERS (CCs)**
>
> - The Trial CC, working within a network or specific trial, is a vital link between all committees overseeing the trial and the investigators and participants at the clinical sites.
> - The CC facilitates numerous important tasks in addition to data collection and site monitoring that need to be completed before, during, and after the study has ended.
> - Multiple CCs in different countries or regions may themselves be coordinated by an Oversight CC (OCC).

PROTOCOL FINALIZATION

For some trials it is possible to send the protocol to potential investigators for their comments and input before it is finalized. Investigators may join protocol review committees or be members of the trial Executive Committee/TSC. Increasing investigator input at the early stage, and maintaining this throughout the trial, may help to develop a sense of ownership of the trial, thus enhancing recruitment and maintaining enthusiasm for the trial.

SITE SELECTION

The selection of sites for a trial is a vital step, and consultation with all relevant parties is required. The responsibility for site selection, unless delegated, remains with the sponsor. Site eligibility criteria should be defined early in trial planning to ensure that appropriate sites are selected. Some questions to address include the following.

- Do the planned sites have a suitable patient population?
- Are there specialist care units that this target group attends?
- Is the site staff qualified?
- Does the site staff have all the necessary equipment, space, and time?
- Is there a high incidence of disease, or is it necessary to recruit sites across additional countries with all the benefits and potential challenges that this will bring?

After identification of potential sites, investigators should be contacted to ascertain their interest in the trial. In some instances, it may be necessary for a confidentiality agreement to be signed before revealing any information

> **SITE SELECTION CHECK LIST**
>
> - historical evidence of successful prior trial participation or network membership
> - sponsor recommendations
> - coordinating center recommendations
> - colleague/investigator recommendation
> - review of medical literature
> - professional meetings symposia
> - directory of medical specialists
> - professional society affiliations
>
> **NOTE:** All potential investigators should be checked to insure they are not banned or disqualified from clinical research (for example that they are not on FDA debarment list. http://www.fda.gov/ora/compliance_ref/debar/).

about the IND/IMP or protocol to the investigator. A copy of the protocol/trial synopsis, summary of product characteristics, or Investigator Brochure should be provided, and time allowed for the investigator to review and consider trial feasibility at his or her site.

SITE EVALUATION

Every site will need to be evaluated for a new trial, even if a site has participated in a previous trial within a network. A trial-specific questionnaire should be completed, in writing or by telephone, or (where there is no previous experience of working with a site or investigator) face-to-face at an evaluation visit. The questionnaire evaluates the feasibility of running the trial at the site with respect to the trial requirements (see box for key questions). It is important that all communication between the site and trial CC be documented and kept in the site file (as well as the CC file).

Site Evaluation Visit

For sites with which the sponsor or collaborators have had no prior trial/study experience, a more comprehensive evaluation in the form of an evaluation visit may be required. If, in these circumstances, a visit is not deemed necessary, the reasons for this must be documented in the

> **SITE SURVEY QUESTIONS**
>
> - Protocol requirements: can the site complete required diagnostic or therapeutic procedures?
> - Patient population: does the site have the necessary numbers of the target populations?
> - Recruitment strategy: potential barriers to enrollment? Need for advertisements? Need for translations?
> - Staff resources and qualifications? Backup personnel available? ICH-GCP certifications? Human subject protection (HSP) training completed?
> - Necessary equipment available? Space for visits? Archiving space?
> - Liability insurance?
> - Willingness to attend investigator meetings?
> - Conflicting/competing studies?
> - Lab/pharmacy/emergency procedures?
> - Previous audits and findings?
> - Does the site have access to all source documents (e.g., external lab results) for monitoring/audit purposes?
> - Does the site staff have ready access to a computer workstation for direct electronic data capture and related electronic communications with the CC? Is hardware/software compatible?

evaluation questionnaire, which should still be completed. At the visit, the CC staff responsible for the trial coordination will evaluate the site for suitability to participate in the trial and complete any trial-specific training and certification of site staff needed. All training, whether initial or periodic refresher training, needs to be documented throughout the course of the trial. The TMG may decide on the specific training strategy, depending on the nature and risk assessment for the trial, but the CC implements all training, site monitoring, and other monitoring of adherence to the protocol and GCP, and will be advising site staff on all trial-specific issues throughout the course of the trial.

At the initial site evaluation visit:

- The PI and site staff proposed to work on the study must all be present.
- All elements assessed in the questionnaire must be reviewed and documented.

- Additional issues may also need to be addressed; for example, the investigator may be asked to explain the site's informed consent procedure.
- The evaluation visit may also offer the opportunity to train the site staff on particular issues.

SUBJECT RECRUITMENT PLANS

Recruitment for a trial should be considered from the start of protocol design, and all protocol requirements assessed from the perspective of both patients and investigators. All sites should have a recruitment plan for the trial with, ideally, a minimum recruitment target. It is essential that targets are realistic. For example, a site that commits to recruiting 10 HIV seroconvertors a year when it only sees 3 cases a year is not helpful to the site itself, CC, or trial as a whole. However, after recruitment has started, additional areas of concern may be identified. To the extent feasible, all relevant information about screening and recruitment at sites should be collected and monitored by the CC. This information may be used to identify effective screening approaches and/or may be used to modify subject eligibility criteria.

Additionally, involving national and local advocacy groups and research networks and considering patient registries may also help with recruitment.

In general, a good rule for site planning is to assume that the number consented and randomized will be 20% to 50% of those screened as likely eligible candidates, depending on the rigor of eligibility criteria.

In the United Kingdom, the 1999 *Health Technology Assessment* report[20] made several recommendations for successful subject recruitment in clinical trials that may be worth considering when planning recruitment:

- Screen twice number of required patients.
- Make contingency plans for low recruitment—adaptive trial design.
- Stagger recruitment at sites to ensure even numbers throughout.
- Conduct a pilot study to test that recruitment strategies are adequate.

Hopefully, careful consideration of accrual from the trial design phase will identify and address most obstacles in advance. These barriers can be varied depending on the type of trial and population targeted; but general considerations are described in the following section.

Potential Barriers to Subject Enrollment
Subject Apprehension
For most people, the decision to participate in a clinical trial is not an easy one to make. Subjects may have recently been diagnosed and may not feel ready to make a decision on future treatments at this stage. Subjects may feel reluctant or apprehensive about joining a trial; there may be a fear of being misinformed, worry about receiving a placebo, or concern about being a "guinea pig." The increased numbers of appointments or hospital stays required for a trial may be burdensome. There may be a variety of problems associated with a diverse subject population, involving language, cultural factors, beliefs about medical research, and the appropriateness of available protocols. Specific disease areas may necessitate special considerations—for example, issues of confidentiality in trials of HIV-infected or AIDs-diagnosed individuals.

Different approaches can help minimize participant concerns:

- Training the site to improve initial discussions with the participants.
- Ensuring that the subject information sheet is clear and appropriate to all target groups.
- Considering the use of interactive technology to improve patient understanding of the trial (this may also ensure more committed participants).
- Considering online web forums for patients to discuss trials generally and more specifically.
- Ensuring that updates and results are fed back to subjects during and at the end of trials to encourage understanding and a feeling of participation.

Trial Design: Raising the Profile of Clinical Trials
Difficulties in accruing subjects from certain patient populations—for example, treatment-naïve patients or treatment-stable patients—can arise. Often the solution is to further increase patient awareness of the trial by:

- Organizing public information campaigns.
- Discussing the trial and collaborating with patient groups.
- Producing information leaflets for site-related clinics/practices.
- Having press announcements and listing the trial on the appropriate websites.

Physician Attitudes

When trying to address certain questions in clinical practice, physicians as well as patients may have their own opinions on best practice, which may or may not be supported by clinical evidence. This lack of equipoise will need to be addressed to enable all sites to participate and recruit to a trial. The CC will need to take an active role in reestablishing physician equipoise, so that randomization is seen clinically as ethical, given the current lack of evidence for or against the experimental treatment(s).

Training and discussion with site investigators, attending clinic meetings to present the trial, producing information sheets, and providing regular trial updates can help engage investigators and sites. However, continuous monitoring of recruitment rates will also be necessary to ensure that equipoise persists.

Maintaining Site Enthusiasm

Many large trials are long in duration, and the CC will need to maintain site enthusiasm through the various stages of the trial and through potential staff changes as well.

MEETINGS

Launch Meetings

At the beginning of a trial, a launch meeting is held, where representatives from existing collaborators, recent participating centers, and any interested centers/collaborating groups can get together to discuss the trial. It offers the opportunity to meet the TMG and coordinating center staff, publicize the trial, encourage accrual, remind sites of the important trial questions, and review key aspects of design and conduct. Launch meetings can encourage a sense of community among the disparate groups and sites and offer the chance for additional collaborations to be made. Slides for the meetings can be circulated to participants for dissemination in a center and to colleagues and for use in internal meetings about the trial.

Investigator Meetings/Educational Seminars

To try and maintain enthusiasm, investigator meetings can be held regularly, perhaps based around international or national conferences/meetings. Here representatives from participating sites and consumer advocacy groups can meet to hear updates and presentation of progress concerning the trial, current accrual rates, discussion of known problems, and consideration of solutions. These meetings offer the chance to remind sites of the ongoing importance of the trial and the opportunity for further training on any specific issues that arise. These forums can also highlight new, related research findings that enhance the relevance of the trial.

COMMUNICATION AND PROMOTION

Regular feedback on trials is desirable to both investigators and participants, and there are various approaches that can be employed, depending on the stage and type of trial involved:

- Press releases.
- Protocol circulation to research networks, charities, and patient groups at the beginning and when amendments occur.
- Trial registration with nonmandatory trial listing websites, which can distribute information to the public, possible patients, clinicians, and researchers who may be interested in participating and generally raise awareness of the trial and research goals.
- Online questionnaires/training/videos and/or scheduled "webinar" trainings can be useful for site staff.
- Attendance at national/international conferences to discuss, advertise, and promote the trial by presentation or a poster stand.
- Newsletters/fliers can be used to report the progress of the trial, offer encouragement, remind sites and participants of the importance of the trial, and discuss relevant issues.

CONCLUSION

This chapter has highlighted the major considerations and pitfalls for any potential trial researcher. Each trial is individual and brings with it a myriad of unique problems and solutions that no one chapter or handbook can cover fully.

The most important tool to enable the successful completion of a trial is good, transparent communication with all participating sites and therefore participants:

- Identify the types of sites to be included and, if applicable, any additional countries to be included up front.
- Understand all regulatory and ethical requirements and the associated timelines in all the participating sites and allow equivalence between regulatory bodies and their procedures.

- Establish trial charters and governance committees before the trial commences, and ensure that each committee is made up of relevant, committed members.
- Appreciate each country's legal and regulatory requirements, and agree up front on how to reconcile variations from the host's requirements in order to minimize delays in the trial start-up.
- Employ an organizational strategy that best suits your trial requirements; an approachable, communicative CC will help in all aspects of running a clinical trial.

REFERENCES

1. Guide for GCP: ICH Harmonised Tripartite guide, June 10 1996. www.ich.org
2. Department of Health South Africa. *Guidelines for Good Clinical Practice in the Conduct of Clinical Trials in Human Participants in South Africa.* www.doh.gov.za/docs/policy/trials.
3. Schuman SH, Olansky S, Rivers E, et al. Untreated syphilis in the male negro; background and current status of patients in the Tuskegee study. *J Chron Dis.* 1955;2:543–558.
4. Kampmeier RH. Final report on the "Tuskegee syphilis study." *South Med J.* 1974;67:1349–1353.
5. Stephens T, Brynner R. Dark Remedy—the impact of thalidomide and its revival as a vital medicine; Published Perseus 2001.
6. McBride WG. Thalidomide and congenital abnormalities. *Lancet* (2):1358 (Dec 11) 1961.
7. The DAMOCLES Study Group. A proposed charter for clinical trials data monitoring committees: helping them do their job well. *Lancet* 2004; 365:711–722.
8. DeMets DL, Fleming TR, Whitley RJ, et al. The data and safety monitoring board of acquired immune deficiency syndrome (AIDS). *Contr Clin Trials.* 1995;16:408–421.
9. Ellenberg SS, Fleming TR, DeMets DL. *Data Monitoring Committees: A Practical Perspective.* New York: Wiley; 2002.
10. U.S. Food and Drug Administration. *Guidance for Clinical Trial Sponsors on the Establishment and Operation of Clinical Trial Data Monitoring Committees.* Draft document. http://www.fda.gov/cber/gdlns/clindatmon.pdf.
11. Fisher MR, Roecker EB, DeMets DL. The role of an independent statistical analysis center in the industry-modified National Institutes of Health model. *Drug Inf J.* 2001;35:115–129.
12. Jennison C, Turnbull BW. Interim monitoring of clinical trials. *Stat Sci.* 1990;5:299–317.
13. Meinert CL. *Clinical Trials: Design, Conduct and Analysis.* NewYork: Oxford University Press; 1986.

14. Pocock SJ. *Clinical Trials.* New York: Wiley; 1983.
15. Sydes M, Altman DG, Babiker AG, et al. Reported use of Data Monitoring Committees in the main published reports of randomized controlled trials: a cross-sectional study. *Clin Trials.* 2004;1:48–59.
16. Sydes M, Spiegelhalter DJ, Altman DG, et al. Systematic qualitative review of the literature on Data Monitoring Committees for randomized controlled trials. *Clin Trials.* 2004;1:60–79.
17. DART Trial Team. Fixed duration interruptions are inferior to continuous treatment in African adults starting therapy with CD4 < 200 cells/µL. *AIDS.* 2008;22:237–247.
18. An open-label randomized trial to evaluate different therapeutic strategies of combination therapy in HIV-1 infection design, rationale, and methods of the Initio trial. *Cont Clin Trials.* 2001;22:160–175.
19. INITIO Trial International Co-ordinating Committee, Yeni P, Copper DA, Aboulker JP, et al. Virological and immunological outcomes at 3 years after starting antiretroviral therapy with regimens containing non-nucleoside reverse transcriptase inhibitor, protease inhibitor, or both in INITIO: open-label randomized trial. *Lancet.* 2006;368:287–298.
20. Prescott RJ, Counsell CE, Gillespie WJ, et al. Factors that limit the quality, number and progress of randomized controlled trials. *Health Technol Assess.* 1999;(3), (20). http://www.hta.nhsweb.nhs.uk/fullmono/mon320.pdf

FURTHER READING

DAMOCLES Study Group. Grant A, Altman D, Babiker A, et al. A proposed charter for clinical trials data monitoring committees: helping them do their job well. *Lancet.* 2004;365:711–722.

Ellenberg SS, Fleming TR, DeMets DL. *Data Monitoring Committees: A Practical Perspective.* New York: Wiley; 2002.

Jennison C, Turnbull BW. Interim monitoring of clinical trials. *Stat Sci.* 1990;5:299–317.

Prescott RJ, Counsell CE, Gillespie WJ, et al. Factors that limit the quality, number and progress of randomized controlled trials. *Health Technol Assess.* 1999; (3), (20). http://www.hta.nhsweb.nhs.uk/fullmono/mon320.pdf.

CHAPTER 8

Quality Control and Quality Assurance

FLORA S. SIAMI

This chapter discusses the quality measures that are necessary in every stage of a clinical trial to maintain the scientific integrity, protect the safety and well-being of human subjects, establish reliability of the data, ensure compliance with applicable regulations, and uphold public confidence. The specific quality assurance issue of missing data is discussed comprehensively in Chapter 9.

Clinical trials are the gold standard for obtaining evidence-based information on therapeutic interventions. Failure to plan and implement (i.e., build in) an effective quality program can adversely affect not only the scientific integrity of the trial but also compromise human subject protection and affect public confidence in the reliability and effectiveness of clinical trials within the medical community.

The International Conference on Harmonisation (ICH) Good Clinical Practice (GCP) guidelines serve as the roadmap to assure quality.[1] This roadmap is even more critical with the changing landscape of clinical trials, including global expansion, participation of vulnerable subjects (e.g., pediatrics, pregnant women), number of sites per trial, number of subjects per site, as well as expansion of investigator pool and new entities (e.g., site management organizations, patient recruitment firms). Thus, quality must be built into the clinical trial process from the beginning.

ICH defines *quality control* (QC) as "the operational techniques and activities undertaken within the quality assurance system to verify that

---

Quality is the backbone of any clinical trial and serves as a cornerstone of clinical trial success.

the requirements for quality of the trial-related activities have been fulfilled."[1] These are the operational checks to ensure compliance. Examples of QC activities include review process for protocol development, double-data entry of paper case report forms, or site monitoring for source document verification.

ICH defines *quality assurance* (QA) as "all the planned and systematic actions that are established to ensure that the trial is performed and the data are generated, documented (recorded), and reported in compliance with Good Clinical Practice (GCP) and the applicable regulatory requirements."[1] This is the mechanism for the systematic, independent examination (audit) of clinical trial activities and documents, and the corrective and preventive action (CAPA) process. Examples of QA activities include training, site audits, and defining process (e.g., statistical analysis plan). Quality should be built into the clinical trial life-cycle. Key components of the QA plan are noted in Table 8.1.

Table 8.1	Elements of a Quality Assurance Plan
Detection Mechanisms	
Central data monitoring (e.g., DSMB or adjudication) Routine on-site visits Remote monitoring Statistical monitoring Audits Site performance metrics Quality control (validation checks, double data entry)	
Corrective Actions	
Correct errors found Retrain investigator and study staff Implement procedures to prevent future errors	
Preventive Actions	
Concise protocol and manual of operations CRFs designed to collect only essential elements Pretest or pilot testing of CRFs and procedures Site monitoring plan Quality control mechanisms Change control for document management	

Errors in the design, conduct, recording (data collection), analysis or reporting of a clinical trial have the potential to affect not only the rights, safety, and well-being of the trial subjects but also the credibility of the trial results.[2] Due diligence in trial monitoring is an integrated process that plays a crucial role in eliminating these errors—whether systematic, random, or fraudulent; it begins with oversight of protocol design and is continued through publication of results.[3] The quality plan is a collaborative effort across all functional areas that defines measurement tools to determine compliance. The trial governance should have standard operating procedures (SOPs) in order to establish the clinical trial execution and compliance expectations.

SITE TRAINING

Education is paramount to establishing standards and improving quality. Site selection (mentioned in Chapter 7) is the opportunity to identify qualified, experienced investigators in not only the therapeutic area but also in clinical research. In most instances, site selection is based upon not only the curriculum vitae of the investigators but also a qualification visit to assess the capabilities and quality of the site and study personnel. The United States' Federal Wide Assurance (FWA) number for local Institutional Review Boards/Ethics Committees (IRBs/ECs) and certification in human subject protection training for investigators and site study staff serve as quality measures for site selection. Typically, an informed consent template is also provided to sites by the coordinating center to serve as a standardized element for the protection of human subjects, including privacy and confidentiality. In addition, investigator kick-off or launch meetings (see Chapter 7) are the ideal opportunity to train sites in a standardized format to ensure quality data collection and compliance. Other training tools—such as the investigator's brochure, manual of operations, case report form (CRF) guides, and investigational product accountability procedures—serve as quality checkpoints to ensure standardization. Good clinical practice checklists for informed consent (critical elements), tracking logs for IRB submissions and adverse event (AE) reporting, screening and enrollment logs for consented subjects, and site signature logs for delegation of duties also serve as resources for ensuring quality.[4]

> Site training is a dynamic process that should be continued throughout the trial life cycle.

Table 8.2 Training Approaches for Clinical Trials

	Pros	Cons
In-person group training	• Same information is disseminated to all participants at the same time by all key trainers	• Expensive • Requires coordination of schedules
In-person site training	• Same information is disseminated to all site personnel • Trains additional site personnel who did not attend the investigator meeting (e.g., lab tech, pharmacist, subinvestigators)	• Travel costs • Requires coordination of schedules • Not all trainers are present, only the CRA
Webinar	• Relatively inexpensive • Can accommodate large groups of people • Same information is disseminated	• Does not have same interpersonal rapport • Limited access to trainer(s)
Self-directed	• Inexpensive • Time accommodates participants' schedule • Can be performed in modules rather than all at once	• Cannot ensure total understanding of participant • Unable to ask questions of trainer • No interpersonal rapport
Telephone	• Inexpensive • One-on-one connection • Personalized to meet the needs of the participant	• No visual aids • Participant can be easily distracted

There are several different methods for training (Table 8.2) that can be used to accommodate time, resources, and budget. In-person group training, such as investigator meetings, is usually best because it ensures that all participants are receiving the same information in the same manner, including any question-and-answer sessions. Training at the site, at a site initiation visit, for example, is also effective because it ensures that all site personnel are receiving the information in a consistent manner. However, due to travel costs and personnel availabilities, in-person training may not always be feasible. In this case, webinars are a great interactive alternative. At webinars, participants are both on the telephone and in front of a computer screen. The trainer controls the screen and the presentation, while the participants can ask questions via telephone or computer in real-time. Training can also be self-directed or performed via telephone, but this is routinely used best as a retraining or refresher tool rather than first-time training. Self-directed training allows the participant to schedule the session at a convenient time, and the presentation progresses forward at the speed of the participant. Questions are generally asked at the end of self-directed training in order to establish understanding of the materials.

SITE MONITORING

Each trial should establish a written site monitoring plan that includes the scope and frequency of routine site monitoring visits as well as guidelines for handling suspicious practices or misconduct in data collection.[5] Once the trial has begun patient recruitment, routine site monitoring visits allow for quality control of regulatory compliance, protocol adherence, source document verification (SDV), adverse event reporting, and query resolution.

However, on-site monitoring is costly and can be inefficient for the identification of errors most likely to compromise patient safety or bias study results.[2] Alternatives to on-site monitoring could include remote monitoring or statistical monitoring (Table 8.3). In *remote monitoring*, the site sends copies of source documents for patients participating in a trial, via mail or fax, to the monitor (e.g., the coordinating center or

Routine monitoring allows for quality assurance throughout the trial.

Table 8.3 Approaches to Site Monitoring

	Pros	Cons
On-site routine monitoring	• Able to perform SDV • Able to perform retraining on the spot • Interpersonal rapport	• Travel costs • Resource utilization • Requires coordination of schedules
Remote monitoring	• Relatively inexpensive • Does not rely on PI schedule • Determines overall compliance for site	• Limited SDV • De-identified source documents may be mislabeled
Statistical monitoring	• Able to find aberrant findings or outliers • Inexpensive • Does not rely on PI schedule • Real-time/on-demand • Generates second-level queries • Captures inter-form data inconsistencies	• Unable to compare with source documents • Unable to determine if real value versus typographical error • Interpersonal relationship restricted • Retraining by telephone or self-directed

contract research organization) after de-identifying the source documents and adding the unique trial patient identification number on each page. The CC/CRO then reviews the de-identified source documents with the data entered into the database. Remote monitoring is ordinarily used on a sample of patients and limited to source document verification of critical elements such as eligibility criteria (inclusion/exclusion) and outcomes or endpoints. *Statistical monitoring* involves running many statistical programs against the clinical trial database to identify outliers, missing or nonsensical data. Statistical monitoring is able to identify trends that are site-specific or patient-specific for further investigation. It is imperative that each clinical trial conduct a risk-based assessment to identify the optimal monitoring method(s), by considering the available resources, the likely sources for error, and the consequences to trial subjects and study validity.

Data monitoring by an independent Data Safety and Monitoring Board (DSMB) or Data Monitoring Committee (DMC) also serves to provide periodic quality checkpoints for safety and continuous quality improvement (CQI). The Clinical Events Committee (CEC) serves to assess trial endpoints and study outcomes in an independent standardized procedure using standardized event definitions.

Formal metrics—such as accrual, follow-up compliance, and missing data rates—are also effective tools in monitoring site compliance.

SITE AUDITING

As a rule, site audits utilize a risk-based approach for acceptable levels of variation that would not affect reliability. Site audits performed by the sponsor, coordinating center, or delegated third-party, are performed using a predefined algorithm in identifying sites that exceed acceptable levels of variation. Thus site audits can be performed (i) randomly, (ii) at sites with very high or very low enrollment, (iii) at sites with very high or very low event rates, or (iv) "for-cause" when persistent protocol noncompliance, falsification, or fraud is suspected or documented.

POOR SITE PERFORMANCE

A good communication plan can help prevent poor performance, which jeopardizes the scientific integrity and credibility of a trial. Retraining is often the first response. However, when serious problems are identified, the trial governance may decide to exclude the site data from the overall results and/or terminate the continued participation of a site. If a site's participation is terminated, the trial governance still has several options for obtaining meaningful data. The site may be:

- Completely terminated, meaning that all subject treatment/intervention and all subject follow-up must be terminated and no additional subjects may be enrolled.
- Restricted, meaning that all subject treatment/intervention should be discontinued, all subjects currently enrolled can complete follow-up, and no additional subjects may be enrolled.
- Open for event tracking only, meaning that all treatment/intervention should be discontinued and no additional subjects may be enrolled,

and subjects currently enrolled are *only* followed for vital status and adverse events.

SITE PAYMENTS

Pre-specified milestones *are usually tied* to site compensation. This is an important incentive to ensure high quality and timely data. Standard site contracts typically include a per-subject payment based upon scheduled visit intervals using several factors outlined below:

- The complexity of the protocol.
    Are there a lot of study visits required?
    Are there a lot of study-specific procedures at each visit?
    Is the dispensing of drug or titration schedule cumbersome?
    Is there a need for special equipment?
- The availability of subjects. For example, is this a study of hypertensive patients, where there are dedicated clinics seeing hundreds of patients, or of hemophilia patients, where a clinic will only see one or two patients per month?
- Subject stipends. For example, will subjects be provided a stipend to cover travel costs, complete questionnaires, or undergo study-specific procedures?

Payment is typically made once all case report forms (CRFs) for the scheduled visit interval (milestone) are completed. If electronic data capture is used, data should be entered with all first-level queries resolved. Some trials incorporate a payment schedule for screening as well as non-evaluable (i.e., ineligible) subjects as a quality measure to ensure that sites are motivated to enroll all subjects who prove to be eligible. Some trials may provide additional reimbursement for screened subjects if the trial involves performing a study-specific procedure to determine eligibility. It is customary to withhold a portion of the payments until the end of the trial, after all queries have been resolved, which is also a quality measure. In addition to the per-patient compensation, a separate predetermined fee (usually around $1,500 to $2,000) is paid to cover protocol and ICF

> Payments are an important quality assurance incentive. Per-patient payments should be carefully planned to optimize protocol adherence and timely, quality data.

submission to the local IRB/EC. This fee is usually paid after IRB submission, and *is not* contingent on IRB approval. Some trials also pay a fee (usually around $125 to $150) for every Serious Adverse Event form that is completed and submitted with relevant source documents.

CONCLUSION

A well-designed and implemented quality control and quality assurance plan will help detect problems early and allow for appropriate corrective action. The quality plan should be built into the clinical trial life cycle from inception.

REFERENCES

1. International Conference on Harmonisation (ICH). Good Clinical Practice (GCP) Guideline E6, May 1996.
2. Baigent C, Harrell FE, Buyse M, et al. Ensuring trial validity by data quality assurance and diversification of monitoring methods. *Clin Trials*. 2008;5: 49–55.
3. Knatterud GL, Rockhold FW, George SL, et al. Guidelines for quality assurance in multicenter trials: a position paper. *Cont Clin Trials*. 1998;19: 477–503.
4. Sather MR, Raisch DW, Haakenson CM, et al. Promoting good clinical practices in the conduct of clinical trials: experiences in the Department of Veteran Affairs Cooperative Studies Program. *Cont Clin Trials*. 2003; 24: 570–584.
5. Pollock BH. Quality assurance for interventions in clinical trials. Multicenter data monitoring, data management, and analysis. *Cancer*. 1994; 74:2647–2652.

FURTHER READING

Ogg GA. *Practical Guide to Quality Management in Clinical Trial Research*. Boca Raton: CRC; 2006.
Robinson M, Cook S. *Clinical Trials Risk Management*. Boca Raton: CRC; 2006.
Valania M. Quality Control and Quality Assurance in Clinical Research. http://www.pharmanet.com/pdf/whitepapers/QCQA.pdf. Accessed May 1, 2008.

CHAPTER 9

Quality Assurance: Prevention of Missing Data

JAMES NEATON

DEFINING THE PROBLEM

The validity of prospective studies, including clinical trials, is threatened by incomplete follow-up data collection for the study participants. The consequence of bias—that is, obtaining the wrong answer—resulting from missing data is greatest for randomized controlled trials of medical and public health interventions, because the results from such studies are the basis for approval for new treatments and are largely the basis of policy statements and treatment guidelines developed by professional societies and governments. A recent review found that missing data in randomized trials was a common problem and that often the methods for handling the missing data were inappropriate.[1]

Although numerous analytic approaches have been published for handling missing data in trials, all involve assumptions than cannot be completely verified. For this reason, the *focus should be on the prevention of missing data*. During the follow-up period of trials, quality assurance efforts should be focused primarily on the complete collection of the major efficacy and safety outcomes of interest for the duration of follow-up, in all participants randomized.

Following presentation of key definitions, reasons for missing data are discussed and suggestions for minimizing the amount of missing data during the conduct of the study are given.

DEFINITIONS OF MISSING DATA

A wide variety of terms, many confusing, are used to describe missing data for trial participants after they are randomized.[2] In part, this is because there are many levels of missing data. Items on a questionnaire

> **FIRST RULE FOR SUBJECT FOLLOW-UP**
>
> In order to carry out an appropriate intent-to-treat analysis (i.e., an analysis where all participants and their outcomes are counted according to the treatment to which they were randomly assigned), patients who discontinue treatment must be followed for all outcomes until the planned end of the study.

may be overlooked; a scheduled follow-up visit may be missed; or the participant may move away, limiting his or her ability to attend future follow-up visits for data collection. One of the most confusing matters in trials is differentiating trial participants who no longer can take (or refuse to take) study treatment from participants for whom complete data collection is no longer possible. Data collection does not have to stop (nor should it) for trial participants no longer taking study treatment.

Three terms are defined next that are used in the sections that follow. These are lost to follow-up, withdrawn, and intervention discontinued.

Lost to Follow-Up

Lost to follow-up is defined as a randomized participant for whom an outcome of interest in the trial protocol cannot be observed. In many trials, a participant may be lost to follow-up for one outcome but not another. For example, in a trial of heart failure treatments, a participant's vital status at the end of the trial may be known, but whether he or she has been hospitalized since last seen for a follow-up visit may be unknown. At the end of the trial, this participant would be considered lost to follow-up for an outcome that involved hospitalization, but not for a survival outcome. Similarly, outcomes that require the participant to attend a visit (e.g., exercise tolerance on a treadmill) may be missing, but information on events such as hospitalization and mortality status may be known.

In some trials, the term lost to follow-up is used narrowly to refer only to study participants with unknown whereabouts. We prefer a broader definition as given above. Unknown whereabouts of the participant is but one reason for not being able to observe an outcome of interest. With this definition of lost to follow-up, and since efforts to locate missing participants should continue for the duration of the study, for many outcomes, the percent of participants lost to follow-up is not accurately known until the end of the study.

Withdrawn

Withdrawn is defined as a participant who has chosen to withdraw from all or some of the protocol requirements of a trial. As a consequence of the participant's withdrawal, he or she may be considered lost to follow-up for some outcomes.

As part of the consent process for a trial, participants are told that they may withdraw at any time. For example, the consent for a large HIV treatment trial called SMART that was sponsored by NIH had the following language in the sample informed consent under a subheading titled "What are my rights as a research subject?"[3,4]

> Taking part in this study is completely voluntary. You may choose not to take part in this study or leave at any time.

Language like this is common and is required by Institutional Review Boards, Ethics Committees, and sponsors for most trials.

In some cases, a participant may decide to stop treatment and continue to attend data collection follow-up visits. Some patients may choose to both discontinue treatment and discontinue attendance at protocol-required follow-up visits, but permit regular telephone or mail contact to assess clinical status. Finally, some patients may not want any further contact concerning the protocol, and may insist that their data not be used in any analyses. Minimizing the extent of withdrawal is clearly a goal to minimize missing data.

Caveat

Withdrawal of consent as a reason for loss to follow-up is becoming more common in trials. Cleland, et al. have noted that it is not always clear whether the participant withdrew consent or whether the investigator withdrew the participant from the trial.[5] The latter should be strongly avoided, and the former, as noted, by Cleland et al., might be best documented with a formal withdrawal of consent form.

Intervention Discontinued

Intervention discontinued is defined as a participant for whom the randomly assigned treatment has been permanently discontinued.

The term "permanently" is used to differentiate such participants from those who may have to temporarily interrupt treatment or who do not adhere to the assigned treatment 100% of the time. The assigned intervention may be discontinued for medical reasons (e.g., side effects or use of a contraindicated treatment) or by the participant because he or she no longer wants to participate in the trial.

All Three Types of Loss to Follow-Up

A trial participant may fall into all three categories of lost participants defined above. In most cases, if a participant is lost to follow-up for major outcomes in a trial (e.g., as a consequence of moving away), the assigned intervention has also been permanently discontinued (obviously, this does not apply to a surgical intervention or the implantation of a device). Likewise, if a participant withdraws consent for all trial procedures, he or she is also likely lost to follow-up for some outcomes (i.e., those that have not occurred before withdrawal) and considered as a participant who discontinued the intervention.

REASONS FOR MISSING DATA

In order to develop procedures to minimize missing data, it is important to understand why data are missing in clinical trials. Three general reasons for missing data are discussed in this section. Some protocols stipulate that follow-up data collection ceases completely, or at least partially, when study treatment ceases or changes. In other studies, outcomes are defined that are not ascertainable. Neither of these practices can be endorsed, because as a consequence, an intent-to-treat analysis cannot be carried out for the affected outcomes. The analysis that is carried out as a result of this practice may result in biased estimates of treatment effects and an inadequate database with which to balance risks versus benefits. These are two common reasons for missing data. The third is data that are missing due to poor implementation of the study.

Data Missing by Design

The APPROVe study is an example of a trial in which information on adverse events was not collected after treatment discontinuation. APPROVe was a placebo-controlled study of rofecoxib (Vioxx). The

---

SECOND RULE FOR SUBJECT FOLLOW-UP

As a general rule of thumb, "event-driven" data like mortality and hospitalizations are easier to collect than "visit-driven" data. The former does not require the participant to attend a clinic visit or even be contacted directly. The latter will be missing unless the participant attends a protocol-required study visit.

results of the study led to the withdrawal of Vioxx from the market. In the report of the findings of the study, the investigators note that cardiovascular events were part of a planned assessment of safety and that serious cardiovascular events were adjudicated using prespecified definitions by a committee blinded to treatment group. They also note in the trial report that "data presented include events occurring during treatment and up to 14 days after the last dose of study drug." With their data collection and reporting plan, an intention to treat analysis could not be carried out.[6] Following this report, information on cardiovascular outcomes, occurring after treatment was discontinued, was retrospectively collected.[7]

The practice in APPROVe is unfortunately very common. Many trial protocols stipulate that safety data are not collected following treatment discontinuation or only collected for some short time period, e.g., 14 or 30 days. One reason given for designing studies in this way is that the inclusion of adverse events after treatment discontinuation would dilute the "toxicity" signal. This is often not the case, and Lachin summarizes examples where such a practice would actually lead to a loss of power.[8] For many treatments it is an unreasonable assumption that their effects, positive or negative, are not present after discontinuation.

Caveat
Collection of data, at least on morbidity and mortality, following discontinuation of treatment, does not preclude doing analyses in which these data are not used after treatment is stopped, for example, a nonintent to treat analysis. It is important that at least one analysis be by intent to treat, and if the data are not collected, the analysis is not possible.

Another example of data "missing by design" is the discontinuation of data collection if participants cross over to the other treatment arm. This also makes an intention to treat analysis impossible to carry out.

The COMPANION trial is an example of a study that did that and later changed the procotol.[9] In COMPANION, pacemakers with and without a defibrillator versus optimal pharmacologic therapy alone were

---

THIRD RULE FOR SUBJECT FOLLOW-UP

Treatment comparisons in trials for which outcomes are not collected following the discontinuation of study treatment may be biased and associated with greater variability than planned.

evaluated in patients with advanced heart failure. The primary endpoint of the COMPANION trial was the composite of death from any cause or hospitalization from any cause. In this trial, 26% of patients in the pharmacologic therapy group "withdrew" from the study to receive a commercially available pacemaker implant due to arrhythmia or heart failure. Although about one-half of these patients had experienced a hospitalization event, mortality follow-up was not available for them. In contrast, the "withdrawal rates" for the pacemaker and pacemaker-defibrillator arms were much lower—6% and 7%, respectively. Fortunately the sponsor attempted to reconsent the pharmacologic therapy patients who "withdrew" for event data collection through the closing date of the study. As a consequence of those efforts, the primary endpoint was unknown for 9% of the control patients and vital status was unknown for 4%. The corresponding percents for both device arms were 1%.

These two trials illustrate the importance of planning for data collection of all events for all randomized patients from the outset.

Data Missing by Design Due to How Outcomes Are Defined

Ideally, outcomes in a study—particularly the primary endpoint—should be clearly ascertainable in all participants. A trial outcome may not be ascertainable if the participant cannot attend the follow-up visit because he or she is too sick. For example, the Pimobendam in Congestive Heart Failure (PICO) trial was a 24-week placebo-controlled study of the effect of pimobendam (verus placebo) on exercise duration.[10] The investigators observed that 24-week data on exercise duration, the primary endpoint, were missing for some patients due to death or due to a cardiovascular contraindication. Furthermore, the number and reason for missing the exercise duration data varied by treatment group—the missing data were likely informative. Thus, a rank analysis was conducted, in which deaths and missing data due to cardiovascular contraindications were ranked lower than the lowest exercise time change observed.[11] In general, for trials in which mortality is expected to be high, survival should be incorporated into the primary outcome; otherwise findings may be difficult to interpret.

In some trial protocols, "missing data" is equated with "failure" in order to ensure the primary outcome is ascertainable for all participants. For example, guidance from the U.S. Food and Drug Administration (FDA) for studies of antiretroviral treatments for participants infected with HIV recommends that the primary analysis count deaths, losses to follow-up, or use of new treatments because of toxicities to the study treatment as treatment failures along with virologic failures (the efficacy

> **FOURTH RULE FOR SUBJECT FOLLOW-UP**
>
> Treatment outcomes in a trial that are defined largely on the basis of missing data are not acceptable.

outcome of primary interest).[12] Problems in interpreting complicated composites such as this if all components do not trend in the same direction have been reviewed.[13]

Data Missing Due to Poor Implementation and Ways to Minimize Such Losses

There are several steps that should be taken during the planning and conduct of a trial to minimize missing data (see Tables 9.1 and 9.2). Examples of strategies for minimizing missing data have been discussed by others.[14–17]

In the design, it is a good idea to inflate sample size to account for missing data. The following is a statement from the SMART protocol for which the primary endpoint was progression to AIDS or death:

> Two percent of patients will be lost to follow-up each year. It is recognized that if the loss rate is as high as 2% per year then estimates of treatment differences for major endpoints could be

Table 9.1 Prevention: Minimizing Missing Data at the Design Stage

- Define easily ascertainable endpoints.
- Inflate sample size in anticipation of missing data to preserve power.
- Specify that data collection for efficacy and safety outcomes is to continue for all patients until the end of the planned follow-up.
- Define follow-up schedule to be consistent with standard of care and with wide windows for completion.
- Select sites convenient for study participants and with a track record for following as well as enrolling participants.
- Plan to select participants who understand protocol requirements and can be followed.
- Emphasize the importance of complete data collection during investigator planning meetings and training sessions and set high standards for the participating sites.

> **Table 9.2 More Prevention: Quality Assurance Procedures Aimed at Maintaining Excellent Follow-Up for Ongoing Studies**
>
> - Plan to collect contact information and periodically update it in the event the study participant cannot be located.
> - Provide transportation costs to participants for study visits.
> - Develop reporting systems to provide up-to-date summaries of data completeness, including visit reminders and missed visit reports.
> - Regularly discuss summaries of follow-up visit completeness and missing data with investigators at meetings.

severely biased. (Since the loss rate is approximately the same as the expected primary event rate, small differences in the rate of events that would have been observed among the losses could result in a different finding.) Nevertheless, this conservative adjustment to sample size was made in order to increase power because some losses are inevitable.[4]

Sample size was inflated by dividing the sample size by one minus the fraction of losses expected—approximately 0.85 for SMART as the planned duration of follow-up was 7.5 years.

When a trial is being organized, sites should be chosen on their track record for following as well as enrolling participants. Sites should be in a convenient location for access by study participants. Once sites have been selected, protocols and procedures should be established that enable excellent follow-up. These efforts begin with the informed consent and participant selection process. It is critical that participants understand the study requirements, and that investigators select individuals who can comply with the protocol. During investigator meetings or training sessions, the importance of proper informed consent and minimizing losses to follow-up should be emphasized.

SETTING HIGH STANDARDS FOR THE COMPLETENESS OF FOLLOW-UP BY THE PARTICIPATING SITES

Advocate a goal of zero losses for the primary endpoint (even though this may not be achievable, particularly in a long-term study), and develop monitoring guidelines for the study to ensure that the loss rate is kept at a very low level. For example, the following two guidelines on follow-up completeness were stated in the protocol for the SMART study.[4] If either occurred, consideration was to be given stopping the trial.

- Loss to follow-up: 1 year loss-to-follow-up rate >2.5%, or projected overall 3-year lost-to-follow-up >10% or an absolute difference between treatment groups of more than 7.5%.
- Missed follow-up visits: 3 or more consecutive follow-up visits missed in the 1st year by more than 2.5% of patients, or an annual missed visit rate >10%.

The loss-to-follow-up guideline in SMART was for the primary endpoint, progression to AIDS or death. As noted earlier, the actual loss rate for an outcome variable like this is usually not known until the end of the study. Patients may be temporarily lost, but sites should not give up on locating such patients and trying to ascertain their endpoint status. In SMART, an interim definition of lost to follow-up was used—no contact for 8 months or withdrawal of consent. Such interim definitions can be helpful for monitoring trial progress.

Unless there are good reasons otherwise, windows for follow-up visits should abut one another. For example, if participants are to be seen every 4 months, windows for the visit should be ±2 months so that a participant is always in the window for a data collection visit. Study participants should be reimbursed for travel costs for study visits.

With clearly defined follow-up data collection schedules, sites can be sent reminders for upcoming visits and reminders for when visit windows are going to close. Procedures to "close the loop" on follow-up visits that are missed should be established—that is, there should be no uncertainty about whether a required data collection visit was completed or not. In some trials, investigators are paid on a quarterly basis for "clean" forms completed at follow-up visits. This can be an incentive for getting participants to attend visits and for carefully completing the required paperwork.

FIFTH RULE FOR SUBJECT FOLLOW-UP

Where applicable, follow-up visit and data collection schedules should be consistent with what is normal or standard of care and monitoring guidelines for site performance should be pre-specified.

Missing data before randomization (baseline data) should also be avoided as it limits ability to describe the study population, assess changes from baseline, and carry out subgroup analyses. This can be ensured in some trials by requiring baseline data to be in the database before a random treatment assignment is issued.

Quality assurance begins at the site level. Sites should be provided timely summary reports on the completeness of follow-up visits and the collection of key data items at the visits so that they can closely monitor their own performance and can easily remind participants of upcoming appointments and identify participants who are not attending visits as planned.

Prior to randomization, contact information for participants and for individuals who are likely to know the whereabouts of the study participant should be obtained; this information should be periodically updated.

OTHER METHODS TO MINIMIZE MISSING DATA

In some trials it may be necessary to go to extremes to collect data from study participants (Table 9.3). For example, in a large HIV treatment trial called FIRST,[18] collection of data on CD4+ cell count was considered very important. Thus, a system was set up with a commercial laboratory to enable participants who moved away to have blood drawn and analyzed in several cities across the United States.

In the Multiple Risk Factor Intervention Trial, silent myocardial infarction was determined from a resting electrocardiogram carried out annually and was an important secondary outcome. For participants who could not attend the clinic, home visits were made to record the electrocardiogram.[19]

In some studies, partial data can be collected by telephone. Similarly, if a major outcome for a study is change in a measurement from baseline to a specific time-point in follow-up, have a plan for obtaining measurements either earlier or later than planned if a study appointment cannot be kept.

SIXTH RULE FOR SUBJECT FOLLOW-UP
Some data is usually better than no data.

Table 9.3	When All Else Fails

- Telephone data collection or partial data collection visits
- More convenient locations for data collection
- Home visits
- Central data sources to check vital status

Central data sources like the National Death Index and Social Security Administration database can be used to confirm vital status in the United States. Most other countries also have central death registries. In the United States, the Social Security number, study participant's last name, and date of birth are key identifying factors that need to be collected to use these databases. These identifying data have been collected with a separate consent in several HIV studies, and over 90% of participants consent to the use of their identifying information for this purpose.

CONCLUSION

- *A goal of no losses should be set at the beginning of a study.* Good follow-up, a trial characteristic that is important for accurately quantifying the benefits and risks of treatment, has not received sufficient attention. Goals should be set high. Various estimates have been given as to what percent lost to follow-up is considered tolerable. These range from 5% to 20%.[14] Matts et al. showed that "tolerable" loss levels depend on the rate of the outcome of interest and the direction of differential losses by treatment group.[20] For sample size, a conservative lost rate (i.e., a lost rate that is higher than one would want because of bias concern) should be set to ensure power is adequate. In recognition of the importance of excellent follow-up, guidelines for stopping the study if missing data are excessive should be stated.
- *Prevention is always better than attempting a cure.* We must shift our focus from design and analytic methods aimed at coping with poor follow-up to methods for improving follow-up during the conduct of clinical trials. In 1953, Bradford Hill stated that "one must go seek more facts, paying less attention to technics of handling the data, and far more to the development and perfection of methods for obtaining them."[21] Fifty years later, an editorial noted that the bias resulting from poor follow-up in clinical trials cannot be corrected in the analysis, and widely used analytic procedures to do so depend on assumptions that are usually not defensible.[22]

This old and continuing advice is important to heed. Plans for preventing missing data are critical components of trial designs and implementation plans.

REFERENCES

1. Wood AM, White IR, Thompson SG. Are missing outcome data adequately handled? A review of published randomized controlled trials in major medical journals. *Clin Trials.* 2004;1:368–376.
2. Meinert CL. Beyond CONSORT: need for improved reporting standards for clinical trials. *JAMA.* 1998;279:1487–1489.
3. The Strategies for Management of Antiretroviral Therapy (SMART) Study Group. CD4+ count-guided interruption of antiretroviral treatment. *N Engl J Med.* 2006;355:2283–2296.
4. Strategies for Management of Antiretroviral Therapy (SMART) Protocol. Bethesda, MD: National Institutes of Health. 2003. http:///www/insight.ccbr.umn.edu.
5. Cleland JGF, Torp-Pederson C, Coletta AP, et al. A method to reduce loss to follow-up in clinical trials: informed, withdrawal of consent. *Euro J Heart Fail.* 2004;6:1–2.
6. Bresalier RS, Sandler RS, Quan H, et al. Cardiovascular events associated with rofecoxib in a colorectal adenoma chemoprevention trial. *N Engl J Med.* 2005;352:1092–1102.
7. Bresalier RS, Sandler RS, Quan H, et al. Cardiovascular events associated with rofecoxib in a colorectal adenoma chemoprevention trial. *N Engl J Med.* 2005;352:1092–1102.
8. Lachin JM. Statistical considerations in the intent-to-treat principle. *Cont Clin Trials.* 2000;21:167–189.
9. Bristow MR, Saxon LA, Boehmer J, et al. Cardiac-resynchronization therapy with or without an implantable defibrillator in advanced chronic heart failure. *N Engl J Med.* 2004;350:2140–2150.
10. The Pimobendan in Congestive Heart Failure (PICO) investigators. Effect of pimobendan on exercise capacity in patients with heart failure: main results from the Pimobendan in Congestive Heart Failure (PICO) trial. *Heart.* 1996;76:223–231.
11. Lubsen J, Kirwan B. Combined endpoints: can we use them? *Stat Med.* 2002;21:2959–2970.
12. Guidance for Industry. Antiretroviral drugs using plasma HIV RNA measurements—clinical considerations for accelerated and traditional approval. U.S. Department of Health and Human Services. Food and Drug Administration. Center for Drug Evaluation and Research (CDER), October 2002.
13. Neaton JD, Gray G, Zuckerman BD, et al. Key issues in endpoint selection for heart failure trials: composite endpoints. *J Card Fail.* 2005; 11:567–575.

14. Schulz KF, Grimes DA. Sample size slippages in randomized trials: exclusions and the lost and wayward. *Lancet.* 2002;359:781–785.
15. Sprague S, Leece P, Bhandari M, et al. Limiting loss to follow-up in a multicenter randomized trial in orthopedic surgery. *Cont Clin Trials.* 2003; 24:719–725.
16. Wisniewski SR, Leon AC, Otto MW, et al. Prevention of missing data in clinical research studies. *Biol Psychiatry.* 2006;59:997–1000.
17. Woolard RH, Carty K, Wirtz P, et al. Research fundamentals. Follow-up of subjects in clinical trials: addressing subject attrition. *Acad Emerg Med.* 2004; 11:859–866.
18. MacArthur RD, Novak RM, Peng G, et al. A comparison of three highly active antiretroviral treatment strategies consisting of non-nucleoside reverse transcriptase inhibitors, protease inhibitors, or both in the presence of nucleoside reverse transcriptase inhibitors as initial therapy (CPCRA 058 FIRST Study): a long-term randomized trial. *Lancet.* 2006;368:2125–2135.
19. Multiple Risk Factor Intervention Trial Research Group. Multiple Risk Factor Intervention Trial (MRFIT): coronary death, non-fatal myocardial infarction, and other clinical outcomes. *Am J Cardiol.* 1986;58:1–13.
20. Matts JP, Launer CA, Nelson ET, et al. A graphical assessment of the potential impact of losses to follow-up on the validity of study results. *Stat Med.* 1997;16:1943–1954.
21. Hill AB. Observation and experiment. *N Engl J Med.* 1953;248:995–1001.
22. Ware JH. Interpreting incomplete data in studies of diet and weight loss. *N Engl J Med.* 2003;348:2136–2137.

FURTHER READING

Cleland JGF, Torp-Pederson C, Coletta AP, et al. A method to reduce loss to follow-up in clinical trials: informed, withdrawal of consent. *Euro J Heart Fail.* 2004;6:1–2.

Lachin JM. Statistical considerations in the intent-to-treat principle. *Cont Clin Trials.* 2000;21:167–189.

Matts JP, Launer CA, Nelson ET, et al. A graphical assessment of the potential impact of losses to follow-up on the validity of study results. *Stat Med.* 1997;16:1943–1954.

Wood AM, White IR, Thompson SG. Are missing outcome data adequately handled? A review of published randomized controlled trials in major medical journals. *Clin Trials.* 2004;1:368–376.

Woolard RH, Carty K, Wirtz P, et al. Research fundamentals. Follow-up of subjects in clinical trials: addressing subject attrition. *Acad Emerg Med.* 2004;11:859–856.

SECTION III

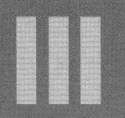

The Future

CHAPTER 10

Surrogate Endpoints

ROBERT FIORENTINO

Pivotal trials are intended to determine the effect of treatment on a clinical endpoint of interest. The less frequently such endpoints occur, or the longer they take to occur, the more expensive the trial and the longer the trial duration. In order to more efficiently perform trials, endpoints predictive of the clinical endpoint that occur sooner or more frequently are sometimes substituted for the clinical endpoint of interest. These are called surrogate endpoints. An example would be the use of blood pressure rather than stroke in a trial of an antihypertensive drug intended to reduce the risk of stroke. Surrogate endpoints are the subject of this chapter.

BACKGROUND

Although there is no universally accepted definition of a surrogate endpoint, many have been offered. For example, Temple[1] proposed that "a surrogate endpoint of a clinical trial is a laboratory measurement or a physical sign used as a substitute for a clinically meaningful endpoint that measures directly how a patient feels, functions or survives." Other definitions focus on the relationship between the surrogate and the clinical endpoint that it predicts; for example, "a surrogate endpoint is expected to predict clinical benefit (or harm or lack of benefit or harm) based on epidemiologic, therapeutic, pathophysiologic, or other scientific evidence."[2]

There also is no standardized classification system for types of surrogate endpoints, although they could effectively be classified as *biological*, *clinical*, or *mechanical*. Examples of biological surrogates include serum LDL cholesterol levels in cardiology trials or HIV RNA levels in AIDS trials. Potentially, they may also include measures of pathologic or physiologic function. An example of a clinical surrogate for oncology trials is measure of tumor response, based on MRI or CT scans. Mechanical surrogates, specific to medical devices, are measures of device function that may predict long-term safety and performance.

SCOPE

Beyond efforts to more precisely define and classify surrogates, there have been considerable efforts to explore *statistically* the necessary relationship between a surrogate endpoint and the clinical endpoint that it is intended to predict. The ability of a surrogate to replace a clinical endpoint in a clinical trial rests on the surrogate not only correlating with the clinical outcome but actually predicting it with a high level of certainty. Regarding the term "prediction," it should be noted that a change in a surrogate does not necessarily precede the actual clinical event in every subject. For instance, although lower blood pressure may be used as a surrogate for a lower risk of stroke in antihypertensive trials, subjects can suffer strokes at any time point along their treatment course, even before meaningful reductions in blood pressure have been achieved by therapy. Likewise, subjects who "fail" to respond to the treatment based on measurement of the surrogate may never experience the clinical event in the course of the trial. In this respect, even though clinical trials may use the surrogate as a "predictive" assessment of a clinical outcome, for individual patients enrolled in the trial this may not hold true. It is therefore important to understand both the statistical relationship and pathophysiologic correlation between a surrogate and its associated clinical endpoint prior to incorporating them into prospective clinical trials.

Prentice[3] published a landmark paper in 1989 proposing formal criteria required to validate a potential surrogate. These have since come to be referred to as the "Prentice criteria" in the literature. These criteria sought to lay out the relationship between the treatment, surrogate endpoint, and clinical outcome in strictly statistical terms. Following this paper, there was some debate surrounding the stringency of the Prentice criteria[4] and whether these criteria could be fulfilled or were even necessary. Further exploration of the Prentice criteria examining the statistical relationship between surrogates and clinical outcomes was carried out in the 1990s, notably by Freedman et al.[5] and Buyse and Molenberghs.[6]

As Fleming and DeMets[7] have pointed out, the Prentice criteria require that the surrogate be both a correlate of the true clinical outcome and also capture the net effect of treatment on the clinical outcome.

However, in practice it can be difficult to establish that a given surrogate captures the net treatment effect on the clinical outcome. This could be because of insufficient scientific knowledge about the biological pathways involved in the disease process. In such a case, the treatment may affect the clinical outcome through a disease pathway unrelated to the surrogate, resulting in the surrogate failing to "capture" the overall treatment effect on that outcome. Difficulty in establishing a surrogate may also arise if there is an insufficient number of patients enrolled in a randomized controlled trial (RCT) for robust statistical characterization of the surrogate. In some cases, meta-analyses of multiple RCTs may be needed to provide adequate information to validate the surrogate endpoint. This is perhaps one of the more widely adopted strategies to validate surrogate endpoints and can include the use of either trial- or patient-level data. Daniels and Hughes[8] have evaluated the association between the difference in treatment effects on a clinical outcome and the difference in treatment effects on the potential surrogate over a range of trials as a means to evaluate a potential surrogate. They specifically applied their methodology to HIV trials to evaluate CD4+ T-cell counts as a potential surrogate for treatment effects on AIDS or death.

Given that this area is an active area of research, a number of strategies have been proposed to establish that the effect of treatment on a potential surrogate outcome correlates with the treatment effect on the clinical endpoint. Such work aims to identify methods through which meaningful conclusions can be drawn regarding the effect of an intervention on the true clinical endpoint of interest.[9]

The severity of the possible consequences of using an inappropriately validated surrogate endpoint has been illustrated by trials that have employed surrogates that inadequately defined the disease pathway. If there are other disease pathways that are not mediated through the surrogate and it is unclear which pathway the treatment or intervention affects, that surrogate becomes much less useful. For instance, there are many ways for a subject in any given clinical trial to experience a failure, such as death. In fact, it is entirely plausible that the treatment or intervention itself may cause subjects to be at a higher risk of death in a manner that is wholly unanticipated. Because drugs interact with the human body in unpredictable ways, relying on a specific biological marker may fail to capture the overall impact of the treatment on the patient.

Figure 10.1 illustrates situations in which a surrogate may fail to predict clinical benefit.

Although surrogates have the potential to reduce the duration and expense of clinical trials, they should be used with caution in pivotal

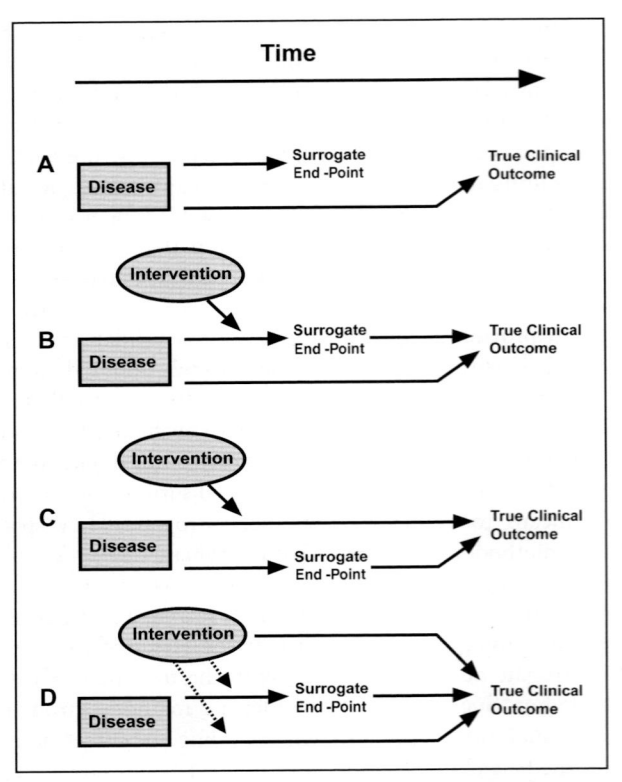

FIGURE 10.1 Reasons for failure of surrogate endpoints. A. The surrogate is not in the causal pathway of the disease process. B. Of several causal pathways of disease, the intervention affects only the pathway mediated through the surrogate. C. The surrogate is not in the pathway of the intervention's effect or is insensitive to its effect. D. The intervention has mechanisms of action independent of the disease process. Dotted lines = mechanisms of action that might exist.[7]

(Phase III) trials. The primary goal of a pivotal trial is to establish that a treatment has a clinically meaningful benefit, and basing the conclusions of the study solely on the evidence provided by a surrogate can be both misleading and even harmful. There are a number of trial examples that erroneously relied on a surrogate outcome as a substitute for a true clinical benefit, one of which will be discussed below.

The Cardiac Arrhythmia Suppression Trial (CAST)[10–12] was an NIH-sponsored study that was designed to test the hypothesis that pharmacologic suppression of asymptomatic arrhythmias in patients who had a previous myocardial infraction (MI) would reduce their risk of death. For years prior to this trial it was observed that post-MI patients with a specific type of arrhythmia were at a higher risk of death compared to patients without them. The belief at the time was that suppression of these arrhythmias using "anti-arrhythmic" drugs would prevent their death. In fact, the effectiveness of anti-arrhythmic drugs prior to the CAST trial was primarily determined by their ability to suppress arrhythmias. This widely held belief resulted in the CAST trial using suppression of arrhythmias as a surrogate for clinical benefit, or reduction in mortality. The three anti-arrhythmic drugs evaluated in the trial (encainide, flecainide, and moricizine) had been FDA-approved for their ability to suppress arrhythmias.

The findings of the CAST study were alarmingly surprising in that the risk of death in the anti-arrhythmic arm of the trial was actually higher than in the placebo arm even though the surrogate endpoint showed a treatment effect. This was because although the anti-arrhythmic drugs did suppress asymptomatic arrhythmias, they also increased arrhythmic death. Clearly, reliance on arrhythmia suppression alone as a surrogate did not capture the net overall benefit or, in this case, harm of this treatment strategy in this specific patient population.

IMPLEMENTATION

It should be noted that despite the above caveats, surrogates have been accepted by regulatory bodies in a number of specific circumstances, including HIV trials, as discussed previously. As noted in an FDA guideline,[13] the feasibility of using HIV RNA levels as a surrogate endpoint was discussed by a public advisory committee that evaluated the relationship between treatment-induced changes in HIV RNA and clinical endpoints. This public discussion of the available clinical data in the presence of regulatory scientists was an important means by which this surrogate could be accepted by the medical community and the FDA. The decision to rely upon a surrogate rather than a clinically meaningful endpoint should not be at the expense of sound scientific investigation and established regulatory principles.

CONCLUSION

Surrogate endpoints can provide significant advantages in time and cost of clinical trials, but can also be double-edged swords. Even within successful trials using an established, validated surrogate, long-term follow-up can be important to further characterize the durability of the treatment effect and net clinical benefit.

Such long-term follow-up does not necessarily include additional randomized controlled trials. As discussed in the next chapter, registries can have distinct advantages when trying to understand treatment effects outside of RCTs.

REFERENCES

1. Temple RJ. A regulatory authority's opinion about surrogate endpoints. In: Nimmo WS, Tucker GT, eds. *Clinical Measurement in Drug Evaluation.* New York: Wiley; 1995:1–22.
2. Biomarkers Definitions Working Group. Biomarkers and surrogate endpoints: preferred definitions and conceptual framework. *Clin Pharmacol Ther.* 2001;69:89–95.
3. Prentice RL. Surrogate endpoints in clinical trials: definition and operational criteria. *Stat Med.* 1989;8:431–440.
4. Fleming TR, Prentice RL, Pepe MS, et al. Surrogate and auxiliary endpoints in clinical trials, with potential applications in cancer and AIDS research. *Stat Med.* 1994;13:955–968.
5. Freedman LS, Graubard BI, Schatzkin A. Statistical validation of intermediate endpoints for chronic diseases. *Stat Med.* 1992;11:167–178.
6. Buyse M, Molenberghs G. Criteria for the validation of surrogate endpoints in randomized experiments. *Biometrics.* 1998;54:1014–1029.
7. Fleming TR, DeMets DL. Surrogate end points in clinical trials: are we being misled? *Ann Intern Med.* 1996;125:605–613.
8. Daniels MJ, Hughes MD. Meta-analysis for the evaluation of potential surrogate markers. *Stat Med.* 1997;16:1965–1982.
9. Weir CJ, Walley RJ. Statistical evaluation of biomarkers as surrogate endpoints: a literature review. *Stat Med.* 2007;26:1415–1416.
10. Echt DS, Liebson PR, Mitchell LB, et al. Mortality and morbidity in patients receiving encainide, flecainide, or placebo. The Cardiac Arrhythmia Suppression Trial. *N Engl J Med.* 1991;324:781–788.
11. Cardiac Arrhythmia Suppression Trial-II investigators. Effect of antiarrhythmic agent moricizine on survival after myocardial infarction: the Cardiac Arrhythmia Suppression Trial-II. *N Engl J Med.* 1992;327:227–233.
12. Cardiac Arrhythmia Suppression Trial (CAST) investigators. Preliminary report: effect of encainide and flecainide on mortality in a randomized trial of arrhythmia suppression after myocardial infarction. *N Engl J Med.* 1989; 321:406–412.
13. Guidance for Industry Antiretroviral Drugs Using Plasma HIV RNA Measurements—Clinical Considerations for Accelerated and Traditional Approval. http://www.fda.gov/cder/guidance/3647fnl.pdf.

CHAPTER 11

Registries

HESHA DUGGIRALA

Registries can serve as an important complement to randomized controlled trials (RCTs). They can be used to collect data in a comprehensive manner with few excluded patients and therefore yield results that may be more generalizable to a wider range of patients compared to RCTs. Furthermore, registries can be used where RCTs are not appropriate or practical (e.g., rare diseases) or when RCTs are unethical.[1]

It is important to note that the concept presented here is the idea of registries as a mechanism for performing observational studies. This is different from the concept of a registry as a listing of ongoing clinical trials.[2] Such a clinical trials registry allows professionals to be aware of ongoing trials and updates their status more rapidly and more frequently than using the published literature alone.

BACKGROUND

By definition, registries are listings of all occurrences of a disease, or category of disease, within a defined area. However, in addition to a disease group, registries may also be classified according to treatment. Registries may collect relatively detailed information and may identify patients for long-term follow-up or for specific laboratory or epidemiologic investigation.[3] Population-based registries (encompassing a specific geographic area or other specified type of population) are usually considered to be the most useful type for epidemiologic purposes; clinic-based, disease-specific registries may be used as a source of cases for case-control studies.[4]

Registries can be designed to serve a number of purposes. A registry may be designed to collect hypothesis-generating data to address a specific question, to help to further characterize the long-term safety and efficacy of a treatment, or to characterize the overall public health impact of the treatment on the disease.

Registries can serve as an important mechanism to collect comprehensive information on patients in various treatment classes or disease groups, as well as to study real-world medical practices. Registries can be used for describing the natural history of disease, determining treatment effectiveness, compliance or cost-effectiveness, collecting quality-of-life measurements, or calculating incidence, prevalence, and survival.[4,5]

The level of detail collected can vary greatly across registries, from being a broad "all-comers" population to following highly restrictive inclusion criteria. For the majority of registries, however, the main exclusion criterion is not having the disease or treatment under study. In this situation, recruitment can be fairly broad to allow for studying a wide population.

DESIGN

Registries may be established for a number of reasons, with great variability in their size, scope, and resource requirements, as is seen across the various ongoing registries in existence. The sample size of registries may be large or small. They may target rare or common conditions and exposure, and they might require the collection of limited or extensive data. In addition, the scope and focus of a registry may be adapted over time to reflect updated information, to reach broader or different populations, to assimilate additional data, to focus on or expand to different geographical regions, or to add new research questions. In addition to recruiting new subjects into a registry, information can be transferred into a registry from existing databases, such as demographic information from a hospital admission or discharge, or from medication use logged in a pharmacy database. Disease and treatment information, such as details of the coronary anatomy and percutaneous coronary intervention, can also be found in (catheterization) laboratory information systems, electronic medical records, or medical claims data.[5]

The initial steps in planning a registry should include articulating the purpose and objective(s) of the registry; determining if the data being sought have already been collected elsewhere; deciding whether a registry is the most appropriate means for addressing the research question; identifying the stakeholders; defining the scope of the registry, including the planned representativeness of the target population and the characteristics of the data to be collected; and assessing if the proposed registry is feasible and likely to be successful.[5] Representativeness is an important consideration. In other words, it is important that the study population be reflective of the population to whom the study results will be extrapolated. Registries, by usually having broad enrollment criteria, are often able to represent a broad segment of the general population.

The purpose of the registry should be carefully considered beforehand, since it is important to generate an *a priori* "hypothesis" if there is a question to be answered. Registries may or not include a control or comparison group; however, most do not. If a comparison group exists, it can be an internal, external, or historical control group. An internal control means that a comparison group can be enrolled within the registry itself. External controls would involve identifying a group outside of the registry population with which to compare outcomes. Historical controls are individuals who had the condition, treatment, or exposure under study at a different time.[4] Historical controls are often identified from the published literature. The length of follow-up of the registries is based on the study question. Most registries, such as cancer registries or registries that involve long-term safety or treatment outcomes, must follow patients for several years to gather the necessary data.

There are several biases that may be introduced in a registry that are similar to those seen with other observational study designs. The term "selection bias" refers to situations in which the procedures used to select study subjects lead to an effect estimate in the study that is different from the estimate obtained from the target population.[3] Selection bias may be introduced, for instance, if certain subgroups of patients are systematically overrepresented or excluded from the registry. Channeling bias, also called "confounding by indication," is a form of selection bias in which drugs with similar therapeutic indications are prescribed to groups of patients with differences in preexisting conditions or prognosis. One example would be a study in which physicians systematically prescribe newer treatments more often to patients who have failed on traditional, first-line treatments.[5]

Information bias refers to inaccuracies in data (i.e., data do not represent what they are intended to represent). One example of how this bias can arise is if an investigator interferes with the outcome assessment, either intentionally or unintentionally. A similar type of bias, reporting bias, may occur in registries when adverse events, or the patients experiencing them, are underreported due to concerns by the investigator or event reporter that he or she will be viewed negatively.[5]

It is important to develop a statistical analysis plan (SAP) that prospectively describes the analytical and statistical methods that will be used to analyze the prespecified primary and secondary objectives.

Generally, the SAP for a registry study intended to support a change in clinical practice, such as a safety registry, is likely to be more detailed than the SAP for a descriptive study.[5]

Although the strengths of registries include the ability to collect large amounts of data rapidly, efficiently, and economically, they are subject to limitations found with other types of epidemiologic studies. As described above, establishing and maintaining registries can be a complex undertaking that may require a large investment of resources. In addition, although registries may include many thousands of patients, it is important to understand that they still are never fully representative of the entire population.

REGULATORY PERSPECTIVE

Registries serve some unique purposes for regulatory agencies. Registries may be used to support or complement Phase I/II drug studies, device feasibility studies, and pivotal trials. Registries are important in pivotal trials when RCTs are impractical or unethical. This is exemplified by studies in which patients refuse open surgery if they know there is a less invasive option available (e.g., aortic grafts, carotid stents, etc.).

Postmarket registries are important for studying the long-term safety and effectiveness of regulated products in a real-world setting. Examples of this are the postmarket registries that were established for coronary drug-eluting stents after marketing approval. At the time of the early drug-eluting stent approvals, manufacturers were required to study implantation of the product in at least 2,000 new U.S. patients in the postmarket period. The objectives of these studies, which were based on single-arm patient registries, were to collect safety surveillance and clinical outcomes data for drug-eluting stents used in routine clinical practice. These registries were needed to evaluate potentially less frequent adverse events and device-related problems (including those of its delivery system) that (i) the pivotal trials were not designed to detect, (ii) may have resulted from subsequent changes in the manufacturing process, (iii) would be more likely to occur in a "real-world" than in a controlled clinical trial environment, or (iv) occur after an extended period of time, beyond that covered by the clinical trial. The companies were asked to choose study sites that were representative of the general use of their product in the real world, outside of tightly controlled, randomized trials. This included sites that were geographically diverse, including community-based facilities, as well as clinical centers with low, medium, and high stent implant volumes. In these postapproval study registries, the sponsor is asked to report extensive data on patient history, procedural characteristics, medications, and clinical outcomes. These data are used by the FDA and the manufacturer to help assess whether adverse events occurring in the real world are those that would be expected based on clinical trial experience.[4]

CONCLUSION

Registries are an important complement to randomized controlled trials. They assist in answering clinical questions that may not be feasible, practical, or ethical to answer in a randomized trial setting. However, there are many issues to keep in mind in terms of study design and potential biases when designing or evaluating a registry.

REFERENCES

1. DeLong ER, Nelson CL, Wong JB, et al. Using observational data to estimate prognosis: an example using a coronary artery disease registry. *Stat Med.* 2001;20:2505–2532.
2. Spilker B. *Prospective Registration of Clinical Trials. Guide to Clinical Trials.* Chapter 107. New York: Raven; 1991.
3. Rothman KJ, Greenland S. *Modern Epidemiology.* 2nd ed. Philadelphia: Lippincott Raven; 1998.
4. Brown SL, Bright RA, Tavris DR. *Medical Device Epidemiology and Surveillance.* London: Wiley; 2007.
5. Gliklich RE, Dreyer NA, eds. *Registries for Evaluating Patient Outcomes: A User's Guide.* (Prepared by Outcome DEcIDE Center [Outcome Sciences, Inc. dba Outcome] under Contract no. HHSA290200500351 TO1.) AHRQ Pub. no. 07-EHC001-1. Rockville, MD: Agency for Healthcare Research and Quality; April 2007.

CHAPTER 12

Gazing into the Crystal Ball: The Future of Randomized Clinical Trials

MICHAEL J. DOMANSKI • SONJA M. MCKINLAY • MARC PFEFFER

We believe that randomized controlled trials (RCTs) will continue, into the indefinite future, to be the definitive tool for evaluating the effectiveness, risks, and costs of new therapeutic and diagnostic strategies in medicine. The fundamental reason is that human biology is far too incompletely understood and complex to reliably predict clinical effectiveness of new treatments from first principles. Whether enough could ever be known to obviate the need for direct experimental verification is an intriguing question but not the subject of this text. Although advances in our understanding of genetics and disease mechanisms will progress and thus improve our ability to focus on populations more likely to need treatment and/or to benefit from it, *the RCT will remain the ultimate gold standard for evaluating and actually quantifying the impact of new therapies.*

IS THERE A ROLE FOR OBSERVATIONAL STUDIES?

Observational data are usually easier and less expensive to collect. Why not collect data on patients presenting with a particular disease and then draw conclusions based on the observed effect as they are or are not treated? The obvious objection is that treatment assignment is not randomized, and the inherent biases, which are often unrecognized and/or hard to quantify, may result in outcome differences unrelated to the intervention in question. Controlling for biases analytically only partially addresses the major problem of selection bias. There are likely to be unrecognized (and unrecognizable) biases confounding the findings. Additionally, in the absence of randomization, quantitative differences between treatment groups with respect to risk factors, even ones that are recognized, and the effect of their interactions (frequently not understood at a quantitative level), cannot generally be fully controlled for analytically. This is indeed a fundamental limitation of observational studies, and conclusions about therapeutic utility of a new treatment based on observational data alone should be regarded as tentative, subject to confirmation in one or more RCTs. That "promising" treatment differences in observational data are not consistently confirmed in subsequent RCTs underscores this serious limitation of observational data.

ARE THERE INSTANCES WHEN OBSERVATIONAL DATA PROVIDE A REASONABLE ALTERNATIVE TO AN RCT?

When the natural history of a disease is clear and the effect size is very large, an observational study may be definitive. For instance, widely metastatic pancreatic carcinoma is uniformly and rapidly fatal. A new chemotherapy agent that resulted in even a 30% cure—no evidence of disease at 5 years—does not require a randomized trial to confirm effectiveness.

Another setting in which observational studies appropriately substitute for RCTs is when the event rate is too low for an RCT to be feasible. An example is evaluation of a new heart valve for safety. Current valves have a very low complication rate. To demonstrate equivalence of a new valve with respect to complications would require a huge, and hugely expensive, clinical trial, so large and expensive that no manufacturer would ever undertake such a study. The effect of requiring an RCT for regulatory approval would be to effectively end heart valve improvement. How do we get around this dilemma? In the case of heart valves, the performance with respect to complications is well characterized (much as is the prognosis of metastatic pancreatic carcinoma in the example above). This well-delineated complication rate becomes a reasonable basis for comparison (accepted by the U.S. Food and Drug Administration [FDA]), obviating the need for an RCT. So, while it is customary for clinical trialists to bemoan the very real limitations that attend nonrandomized studies, there is a specific, albeit very limited, role for them.

REGISTRIES

Registries are observational studies with all of the limitations that attend nonrandomized studies. However, registries will continue to serve a number of important purposes.

- They provide essential data, very cost-efficiently, with which to design RCTs, when needed information is too sparse, including identification

> **EXAMPLE 1**
>
> **AN INNOVATIVE USE OF REGISTRIES FOR DEVICE TRIALS:** An innovative illustration of this use is for the design of a Phase II/III RCT for evaluating a left ventricular assist system.[1] A registry of eligible patients on waiting lists for heart transplant, established before randomization, would provide, concurrently, 3 or 4 patients consenting to the trial, of whom 1 would be randomly chosen for the device while the others would be assigned as no-treatment controls. Of course, this type of registry also provides very important comparative data on the generalizability of trial results, given the necessarily small numbers in the trial itself (20 randomized to the LVAS, 60 to control).

of endpoints for effectiveness and/or safety; estimating endpoint rates; defining target patient populations and how to recruit them; and identifying key covariates to include.
- Randomized controlled trials provide an important, typically concurrent, comparative dataset with which to establish the generalizability of trial results arising from a more narrowly defined, randomized patient group. What does this mean? An RCT provides the "answer" for the population randomized, but the question is often whether the randomized cohort is really representative of the more general population of patients with the disease. Registries can often help to address this question because they are usually large samples of the population of interest.
- Without narrowing exclusionary criteria, registries generate data that better define concomitant morbidities of the disease entity than most typical RCTs.
- Registries can also serve as a reservoir of patients for recruitment into a clinical trial. In many cases, a large number of registry charts can be screened for suitability even before any patients are contacted, greatly reducing the work of recruitment.
- They provide direct feedback to participating sites about their practice patterns and outcomes relative to their peers.

EMERGING FACTORS AFFECTING COST AND DURATION OF CLINICAL TRIALS

Although RCTs will remain the basis of evidenced-based medical practice, there are substantial practical and methodologic challenges associated with current clinical trial practice, some of which are considered below. Just because results are derived from an *RCT does not make them definitive.*

Surrogate Endpoints

Large RCTs are increasingly expensive and time consuming. For industrial firms with a limited patent life on their products, every day off the market is expensive, making the cost of a pivotal trial the sum of actual study costs and the revenue that could have been generated by having the product in the marketplace. As a result, being able rapidly to perform the pivotal RCTs that are acceptable to regulatory bodies is a priority. The cost of clinical trials is also an important issue for governmental organizations sponsoring research. Because they generally operate on a fixed budget, the resulting "zero-sum game" means that funds expended on one RCT represent an opportunity cost relative to other research, including other clinical trials. So, shortening clinical trials and making them less expensive is a priority of the entire clinical trials community—especially for their continued utility.[2]

The question is how to do this. For example, if one wanted to design an RCT to determine usefulness of a new antihypertensive drug in reducing the risk of stroke or death, then an RCT with a primary endpoint of stroke or death would randomize patients either to standard therapy plus a placebo or to standard therapy with the addition of the new drug being tested and would require observation over an average of several years to observe sufficient endpoints. For this trial, costs will increase either with every year of observation and/or from the increased number of patients to provide sufficient endpoints. What about using blood pressure as a substitute for stroke or death that could be measured, more than once over a short follow-up of at most 1 year? Costs will be dramatically reduced by length of observation and use of a continuous outcome, measured inexpensively multiple times to increase information. Blood pressure is, in this case, a surrogate outcome, defined as an outcome different from, but predictive of, a clinical endpoint of interest (in this instance, stroke or death).

Why not consider this much less expensive, faster option? There is a well-documented relationship of elevated blood pressure to stroke risk and, from prior trials, a known therapeutic benefit of treating hypertension to reduce the risk of stroke. The problem is the potential for unrecognized drug effects. Although the molecule tested in this example may indeed share the effect of blood pressure lowering with drugs known to reduce blood pressure and with it the risk of stroke, it may also have unrecognized biological targets that mitigate the therapeutic effect or cause harm. This possibility obviates the shortcut: a definitive trial of

> **EXAMPLE 2**
>
> **THE DOWNSIDE OF SURROGATE ENDPOINTS:** An interesting real-world example of the failure of surrogate endpoints comes from the study of drug treatment of ventricular arrhythmias to prevent sudden cardiac death (SCD). Based on sound observational studies in patients with known coronary disease, particularly those with reduced left ventricular function, the presence of frequent ventricular ectopy is a recognized risk factor for SCD. A reasonable hypothesis is that suppression of ventricular ectopy following myocardial infarction might reduce the risk of SCD. Most experts assumed that reducing this ectopy would also improve survival. Indeed, anti-arrhythmics were already incorporated into standard clinical practice. The Cardiac Arrhythmia Suppression Trial (CAST)[3,4] examined this hypothesis. Patients with frequent ventricular ectopy following a myocardial infarction, whose ectopy was shown to be suppressed by then-frequently used anti-arrhythmic drugs, were randomly assigned to anti-arrhythmic drug treatment or to placebo. While the anti-arrhythmic drugs suppressed the ectopy, they also resulted in an increase in mortality. Indeed, today the role of anti-arrhythmic drugs in the prevention of SCD is minimal and we now understand that the alteration in the electrophysiologic milieu produced by these drugs frequently increases the propensity to sustained and fatal ventricular tachyarrhythmias. What was known at the time about ventricular ectopy was a reasonable basis for undertaking the CAST study, and the importance of having a definitive answer to this question is underscored.

therapeutic benefit will require testing the effect on stroke or death, as well as other clinical endpoints indicative of possible harm (e.g., myocardial infarction).

This hypothetical example illustrates a general and fundamental limitation of surrogate endpoints. Identifying a biological target that is therapeutic in no way excludes the possibility of unrecognized harmful targets. At our current level of physiologic understanding, we simply cannot predict all of the potential effects of a drug, and this will not change on any foreseeable time horizon. Hence, the role of surrogate endpoints in Phase III pivotal clinical trials is, at most, limited.

The situation with Phase I and II trials is different. At the end of the Phase I and II day, the question is whether to proceed to a Phase III trial. That is, is there sufficient promise to justify the investment of time and money in a definitive trial with clinical endpoints? Early drug studies are usually undertaken because the effect of a drug on the pathophysiologic pathway of a disease would be expected to have therapeutic value. Thus, demonstration of a drug's effect on the pathophysiology could be pivotal in deciding whether there are sufficient grounds to proceed to an RCT with clinical endpoints. A favorable effect on events in the pathophysiologic pathway would provide proof that the expected mechanism of benefit is operative and would provide evidence for proceeding to a full scale Phase III trial. In the hypothetical example above, proving that the drug is indeed effective in lowering blood pressure in a smaller Phase II trial might be central to a decision to continue drug development. For a drug intended for treatment of cholesterol, a surrogate of LDL-C lowering, or HDL-C raising, might contribute to a decision on whether or not to proceed to a Phase III study.

So the key "take-home" point is that surrogate endpoints will continue to have a role in early clinical testing, but fundamental limitations make them, at most, very limited use in definitive clinical trials.

International Regulatory Burden

As a result of the increasingly stringent regulatory environment (see Chapter 7), some trends are rapidly emerging:

- The advent of clinical trial directives in the European Union (EU) has made implementation of clinical trials in the EU increasingly difficult, and this is unlikely to change in the foreseeable future.
- As a direct result of the first trend, sponsors are looking elsewhere to complete trials in a timely fashion for acceptable cost, notably Eastern European countries (not presently members of the EU), Asian countries (India, China, Singapore, etc.), and Latin American countries (in Central and South America, notably Argentina and Brazil).
- Countries outside the EU and North America are rapidly upgrading their requirements to be consistent with at least the Good Clinical Practice Guidelines, thus lengthening time lags for certifications and increasing cost.

Is this situation likely to improve? In the short-term, the answer is no. If multicountry RCTs continue, and sufficient pressure can be exerted internationally by private sector sponsors and governments, perhaps an international standard for clinical trial regulations could be negotiated (possibly through the World Health Organization) and accepted by participating countries. This process will be slow with no guarantees on uniform acceptance by individual countries.

RANDOMIZED CLINICAL TRIALS IN THE INFORMATION AGE

Most major RCTs are designed to detect small differences in treatment effect. They are necessarily large, expensive, and difficult to recruit for, requiring many sites, frequently in more than one country. This is a particular concern in North America and the EU, where it has become increasingly difficult and costly to recruit sufficient patients. Stated simply, a central issue is how large RCTs can be completed more quickly and inexpensively. The growth of computing power has made possible the essentially instantaneous transfer and analysis of increasingly large amounts of data. The wide dissemination of Internet access, even to individuals in remote locations, is making this power available rapidly to much of the world.

The 21st century is witnessing the continuing rapid expansion of (wireless) electronic communication into everyday life through satellite and cell technology. The current and emerging implementation of the electronic Personal Health Record (PHR), controlled by the record's owner, not just by the medical system, is a key component of the electronic expansion. The use of Internet platforms has the potential to shift the paradigm by which patients in RCTs are recruited and followed. A huge number of subjects can be offered the possibility of entry simultaneously and can have an initial screening for no more than the cost of sending an Internet message. Consent to participate, physical examination, and blood and urine specimens can be obtained using more cost-efficient health care workers who routinely make home visits. Drug and placebo can be mailed to the subject. Follow-up and endpoint ascertainment can be completed by Internet, telephone, and with limited home visits. The high-cost clinical site is thus eliminated and trials would be available to much broader populations not living near a clinical site. The full cost savings, including reduction in recruitment time, have yet to be fully explored. For interventions that are feasible with this approach, the savings are likely to be considerable. Also, because trials would recruit more quickly and reach a broader population, generalizability of results would be immediate.

An additional advantage of the Internet is in the handling of electronically stored personal health records (PHRs). This is a concept that has been on the table for at least the last decade or so, and has been (or is currently being) implemented in various forms in most economically advanced countries (EU, Canada, Australasia).[5] In its ideal form, the PHR is an electronic record owned by the subject (or legal guardian) and is broadly transportable using standardized software and formats. Read or write access to the record would be with the subject's consent. Automatic access could be given to selected care providers and for limited periods, as in RCTs. For the clinical trialist, such records could be electronically interrogated for suitable trial subjects who might then be approached for possible consent to participate in the study. This screening will increasingly be completed by the potential participants themselves, who will also facilitate direct acquisition of trial-specific data from the PHR.

Clearly, these trends will not only eliminate (or drastically reduce) costly site recruitment, but will also eliminate the need for equally costly site monitoring and extensive source verification—particularly when the source is an electronically available PHR!

ARE WE UP TO THE CHALLENGE?

In conclusion, we believe the RCT is very much alive and flourishing, despite continuing concerns. We face an exciting challenge and opportunity in this century to realize the full power of RCTs, cost-efficiently and with enhanced generalizability as well as improved quality. What will be required is a complete rethinking of how we design and implement trials in this expanding electronic era, using new technologies, many of which already exist (Fig. 12.1).

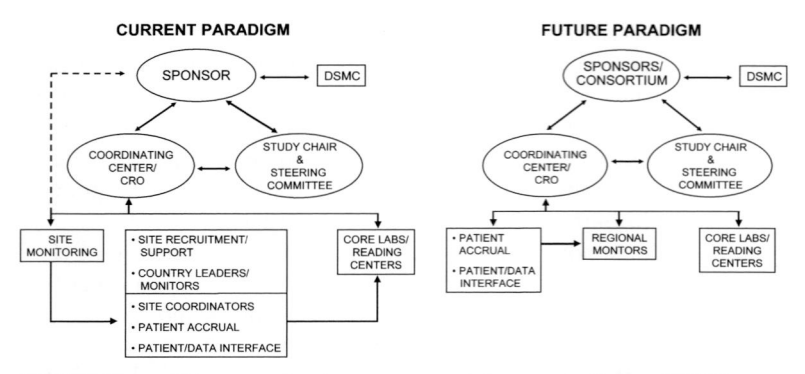

FIGURE 12.1 Diagrams showing current and future paradigms of RCTs.

REFERENCES

1. McKinlay SM, Sleeper LA, Waclawiw MA, et al. Evaluation of an implantable ventricular assist system for humans with chronic refractory heart failure: designing a randomized trial. *Am Soc Artificial Int Organs*. 1995;41:16–22.
2. Ioannidis JPA. Contradicted highly cited clinical research. *JAMA*. 2005; 294:218–228.
3. The Cardiac Arrhythmia Suppression Trial (CAST) investigators. Increased mortality due to encainide or flecainide in a randomized trial of arrhythmia suppression after myocardial infarction. *N Engl J Med*. 1989;321:406–412.
4. Echt DS, Liebson PR, Mitchell LB, et al. Mortality and morbidity in patients receiving encainide, flecainide, or placebo: the Cardiac Arrhythmia Suppression Trial. *N Engl J Med*. 1991;324:781.
5. Anderson GF, Frogner BK, Johns RA, et al. Health care spending and use of information technology in OECD countries. *Health Affairs*. 2006; 25:819–831.

INDEX

Page numbers followed by *f* or *t* refer to figures or tables, respectively.

ACCORD. *See* Action to Control Cardiovascular Risk in Diabetics
Action to Control Cardiovascular Risk in Diabetics (ACCORD), 50
Adverse event (AE), 143
African-American Heart Failure Trial (A-HeFT), 56–57
A-HeFT. *See* African-American Heart Failure Trial
Allocation strategies, 25–26
Alternative hypothesis, 47
Analytic approach and methods
    analysis approaches, 78–90
        alternative statistical approaches, 85–86
        assigned treatment group, null hypothesis, 80
        covariate adjustment, 90
        covariate-adjusted analysis, 84–85
        dilution impact on analysis, 80–81
        face validity, 84
        imaging studies, 88
        important guidelines, 90
        to impute or not, 89–90
        ineligible subject inclusion, 83–84
        interaction test, 86
        ITT, 79–80
        Kaplan-Meier curves, 86
        last observation carried forward, 89
        mean imputation, 89
        missing at random or not, 89
        missing data, 88–90
        multiple imputation, 89
        no study treatment administered, 80–81
        potential bias size, 85
        prespecified definitions, 86
        primary, secondary analytic approach pre-specification, 90
        primary analysis of trial endpoints, 79
        primary and secondary analysis, 79
        a priori adjustment factor selection, 85
        protocol noncompliance, 81–84
        QOL outcomes, 89
        randomization, 90
        randomize missing data, 90
        SHOCK trial, 84
        specified treatment delivery failure, 82, 83*t*
        specimen volumes, 88
        subgroup analyses, 86–88, 88*f*
        subgroup definitions, 86
        subject attrition, 88
        subject exclusion, 90
        treatment arm, subgroup factor interaction test, 87
        treatment crossovers, 80
        treatment dilution, 90

Analytic approach and methods
analysis approaches (*Cont.*)
  trial endpoint secondary
    analysis, 81–85
  worst case imputation, 89
analysis stages, 71–78
  actual *vs.* expected period to
    date, 74
  aggregate *vs.* treatment-
    specific interim analysis,
    77–78
  designated statistician data
    access, 73
  dropping experimental
    arm, 77
  DSMB, 73, 77–78
  DSMB, DMC access, 73
  early trial termination, 77
  eligibility violations, 75
  enrollment feasibility, 73
  event rate, variance
    outcome measure
    estimations, 73
  failure to recruit, failure to
    execute termination, 75
  formal interim trial
    monitoring procedures—
    analysis of variance, 76
  intervention safety, 77
  interventional procedure
    modification, 77
  look and learn, 73
  look and learn trial
    monitoring, 73–75, 74*f*
  new treatment safety, 73
  observed treatment
    difference, 76
  outcome data, interim
    analysis, 77
  post-baseline study out-
    comes, not conducted, 72
  protocol compliance, 73
  protocol violations, 75
  recruitment stage, 73
  restricted access only, 73
  sites, 73–75
  stage I, 72–73
  stage II, 73–78
  stage III, 78
  time periods, 74
  treatment analysis differ-
    ences, data quality review
    exclusion, 71
  treatment arm blinding in
    interim monitoring, 78
  treatment efficacy, 73, 77
  trial design modification, 75
  trial monitoring of variance,
    adaptive design, 76
analytic methods
  categorical, 91
  continuous, 90–91
  time-to-event outcomes, 91–92
choices of significance level, 96
designated statisticians, moni-
    toring board, 72
positive trials, 96
post-hoc power analysis, 96–97
p-Value, 95
reporting results, 93*t*
  absolute rate difference, 94
  categorical outcomes,
    94–95, 94*t*
  continuous outcomes, 92–93
  magnitude of effect and
    variance, 92
  relative difference, 94
  standard error, mean
    difference, 93
  time-to-event outcomes,
    95–97
summary, 97–98

Index

Assigned treatment group, 80
Assmann, Susan, 5–26

Babiker, Abdel, 117–140
Bakobak, 117–140
Belmont Report. *See* Ethical Principles and Guidelines for the Protection of Human Subjects of Research
Bonferroni correction, 50–51
British Medical Journal, 38

CAPA. *See* Corrective and Preventive Action
Case report form (CRF), 148
CATCH. *See* Child and Adolescent Trial for Cardiovascular Health
Categorical outcomes, 94–95
CATs. *See* Clinical Trial Authorizations
CEC. *See* Clinical Events Committee
Child and Adolescent Trial for Cardiovascular Health (CATCH), 62–63
CIOMS. *See* Council for International Organizations of Medical Sciences
Clinical Events Committee (CEC), 146
Clinical Trial Authorizations (CTAs), 121–122
Clinical trial design, 5–26
  allocation strategies, 25–26
  double-blind studies, 20–21
  research question specification, 5–19
    active control, 7–8

binary, 10
clinical relevance, 10
comorbidities, 17
composite outcomes, 12
considerations, 16–17
continuous, 10
count, 10
data collection, 14–15
data to be collected, 10
disease risk, 17
disease severity, 16
eligibility criteria, 16f
equivalence goals, 18–19, 19f
establish difference, 18
goal, 6
how defined, 9
investigational treatment specification, 7
issues, 6
measurement reliability, 10
measurement time period, 14
measurement validity, 10
noninferiority goals, 18
objectivity analysis, 10
ordered categorical, 10
outcome choice, 10
outcome definition, 12–14
outcome measurement, 6
outcome variable types, 10
patient location, 17
placebo control *vs.* no-treatment control, 9
placebo treatment feasibility, 9
placebo treatment risks, 9
population choice, 6
primary outcome, 9
randomization, 17
rate, 10

Clinical trial design (*Cont.*)
  research question
    repeated measure, 10
    sample size implications, 10
    study outcome definition, 9–10
    study phase, 6
    study population, 15–17, 16*f*
    superiority, noninferiority, equivalence, 17–19
    superiority goals, 18
    surrogate outcomes, 10–12
    time period measured, 10
    time to event, 10
    treatment assignment blinding, 9
    treatment considerations, 17
    treatment definition, narrow *vs.* broad, 8*f*
    treatment sensitivity, 10
    treatment strategies, 6
    treatment strategy choice, 7
    unit of analysis, 6, 17
    unit of treatment, 17
  trial design types
    cluster, 24–25, 24*f*
    crossover, 22–24, 23*f*
    factorial, 22, 22*f*
    parallel group, 21, 21*f*
  validity, 20–21
Clinical trials, future considerations, 190
  challenges, 188–189
  costs, duration factors, 184
  examples, 183–185
  information age, 187–188
  international regulatory burdens, 187
  observational studies, 181–182
  registries, 182–184
  surrogate endpoints, 184–186

Cluster trials, 24–25, 62–63
Cochran, Archie, 36
Code of Federal Regulations, 102
Comorbidities, 17
COMPANION trial, 155–156
CONSENSUS II. *See* Cooperative New Scandinavian Enalapril Study II
Continuous Quality Improvement (CQI), 146
Controlled Onset Investigation of Cardiovascular Endpoints (CONVINCE), 108
CONVINCE. *See* Controlled Onset Investigation of Cardiovascular Endpoints
Cooperative New Scandinavian Enalapril Survival Study II (CONSENSUS II), 112
Corrective and Preventive Action (CAPA), 142
Council for International Organizations of Medical Sciences (CIOMS), 92
Covariate adjustment, 90
CQI. *See* Continuous Quality Improvement
CRF. *See* Case report form
Crossovers, 22–24, 53–55, 64–66, 80

DAMOCLES group, 127
DASH. *See* Dietary Approaches to Stop Hypertension
Data and Safety Monitoring Board (DSMB), 54, 73, 77–78, 146
Data collection, 14–15

Data Monitoring Committee (DMC), 73, 124, 126–127, 146
Data Safety and Monitoring Board (DSMB), 146
Declaration of Helsinki, 101–102
Dietary Approaches to Stop Hypertension (DASH), 65–66
Dilution impact, 80–81
DMC. *See* Data Monitoring Committee
Domanski, Michael, 3–4, 181
Double-blind studies, 20–21
DSMB. *See* Data and Safety Monitoring Board
DSMB. *See* Data Safety and Monitoring Board
Duggiralah, Hesha, 175–180
Dunn-Sidak correction, 51

Early trial termination, 77
Effect size, 43, 51–53
Eligibility, 16*f*, 75
Ethical considerations
  background, 102–103
  Belmont Report, 101–102
  Common Rule, 101–102
  confidentiality issues, 108–110
  CONSENSUS II, 112
  CONVINCE, 108
  Declaration of Helsinki, 101–102
  ethics committees, 102, 122–124, 143
  EU, 101
  FDA and, 101–102
  ICH, 102
  informed consent, 103–108, 104*t*

International Conference on Harmonisation, 101
IRB, 102
Nuremberg Code, 101–102
The Oxford Textbook of Clinical Research Ethics, 108
summary, 112
trial futility, 110–112
Ethical Principles and Guidelines for the Protection of Human Subjects of Research (Belmont Report), 101–102
EU. *See* European Union
European Union (EU), 101, 119

Face validity, 84
Failure to recruit, 75
FDA. *See* Food and Drug Administration
Federal Wide Assurance (FWA), 143
Fiorentino, Robert, 167–174
Food and Drug Administration (FDA), 101–102
Friedman, Lawrence, 101–115
FWA. *See* Federal Wide Assurance

GCP. *See* Good Clinical Practice
Geller, Nancy, 45–70
GLMPOWER procedure, 66
Good Clinical Practice (GCP), 141

Hewitt, Catherine, 27–44
Hudson, Fleur, 117–140

ICH. *See* International Conference on Harmonisation
IDE. *See* Investigational Device Exemption
IMP. *See* Investigational Medicinal Product
IND. *See* Investigational New Drug
Informed consent, 103–108, 104*t*
INSIGHT. *See* International Network for Strategic Initiatives in Global HIV Trials
Institutional Review Board(s), 102, 123, 143
Intention to Treat (ITT), 77–80
Interaction test, 86
Interim analysis, 77–78
International Conference on Harmonisation (ICH), 3–4, 49–51, 101–102, 120, 141, 181
International Network for Strategic Initiatives in Global HIV Trials (INSIGHT), 103
Investigational Device Exemption (IDE), 121
Investigational Medicinal Product (IMP), 121
Investigational New Drug (IND), 121
ITT. *See* Intention to Treat

Journal of the American Medical Association (JAMA), 38

Kaplan-Meier curves, 86

Lancet, 32, 38
Large multicenter trials: structure and content, 117–164
Longitudinal studies, 64

MAGIC study. *See* Magnesium in Coronaries study
Magnesium in Coronaries (MAGIC) study, 11, 14–15
McKinlay, Sonja, 3–4, 45–70, 181
Mean imputation, 89
Missing data, 88–90
  APPROVe study, 154–155
  caveat, 155
  COMPANION trial, 155–156
  conclusion, 161
  data missing by design, 154–156
  definitions, 151–154
  FIRST trial, 160
  follow-up completeness standards, 158–160
  intervention discontinuation, 153
  lost to follow-up, 152
  National Death Index, 161
  no losses goal, 161
  outcome design, 156–157
  PICO trial, 156–157
  poor implementation, 157–158, 157*t*, 158*t*
  prevention, 161
  prevention methods, 160–161, 161*t*
  reasons, 154–158
  Social Security Administration database, 161
  subject follow-up rules, 152, 154–155, 157–160
  withdrawal, 153
Multiple imputation, 89

National Death Index, 161
National Institutes of Health (NIH), 109
Neaton, James, 151–164
New England Journal of Medicine, 32, 38
NIH. *See* National Institutes of Health
NQuery Advisor, 66
Null hypothesis, 47, 80

OCC. *See* Overall Coordinating Center
Overall Coordinating Center (OCC), 130
The Oxford Textbook of Clinical Research Ethics, 108

PEACE. *See* Prevention of Events with Angiotensin-Converting Enzyme inhibition
Pfeffer, Marc, 181
Phase I trial, 6
Phase II trial, 6
Phase III trial, 6
Phase IV trial, 6
PICO. *See* Pimobendam in Congestive Heart Failure
Pimobendam in Congestive Heart Failure (PICO), 156–157
Placebo, 9
PLADO. *See* Platelet Dose study
Platelet Dose Study (PLADO), 11, 13–15
Population, 6, 15–17, 175
Post-hoc power analysis, 96–97
Potential bias size, 85
POWER procedure, 66
Prentice criteria, 169

Prevention of Events with Angiotensin-Converting Enzyme inhibition (PEACE), 59–60
Protocol noncompliance, 81–84
Protocol Team (PT), 124, 128–129
PT. *See* Protocol Team
p-Values, 95–97

QOL. *See* Quality-of-Life
Quality assurance, control (QA, QC), 141–149
  CAPA, 142
  conclusion, 148
  GCP, 141
  guidelines, 141
  ICH, 141
  quality assurance definition, 142
  quality assurance elements, 142, 142t
    corrective actions, 142t
    detection mechanisms, 142t
    preventive actions, 142t
  quality control definition, 141
  site auditing, 147
  site monitoring, 145–147
    alternatives, 145, 146t
    approaches, 145–147
    CEC, 146
    CQI, 146
    DMC, 146
    DSMB, 146
    on-site, 145, 146t
    remote, 146, 146t
    SDV, 145
    statistical monitoring, 146, 146t

Quality assurance, control (*Cont.*)
  site payments, 147–148
    CRF, 148
    protocol complexity, 148
    serious adverse event, 148
    subject availability, 148
    subject stipends, 148
  site performance, 147
  site training, 143–145, 144*t*
    AE, 143
    CRF, 143
    ethics committees, 143
    FWA, 143
    IRBs, 143
  SOPs, 143
Quality-of-Life (QOL), 89

r. *See* Effect size
R (software package), 66
Randomization, 4, 27–44, 90
  conclusion, 40–41
  definition, 29
  experimental research, 27–29, 28*f*
  importance, 27–29
  observational research, 27–29, 28*f*
  restricted randomization, 30–32
  sequence protection, 36–40
  simple randomization, 29–31
  subversion (selection bias) risk, 37–40
  techniques
    blocked, 33, 33*f*
    minimization, 34–35, 35*t*
    pairwise, 35
    simple randomization, 32–33
    stratified, 34
  types, 29–32

Randomized Controlled Trials (RCTs), 3, 5
RCTs. *See* Randomized Controlled Trials
Recruitment, 73, 134–136
Registries, 182–184
  background, 175–176
  conclusion, 179
  design, 176–178
  population-based, 175
  regulatory perspective, 178–179
Regulatory agencies, 120–122, 128, 178–179, 187
Repeated measures studies, 98

Sample size determination, 45–46
  accrual rate, 47
  alternative hypothesis, 47
  censored observations, 50, 51
  clinically relevant differences, 47
  competing risk, 50
  composite endpoint, 50, 51
  composite endpoint, ACCORD study, 50
  composite endpoint, ValHeFT study, 50
  continuous measure, 49, 51
  control group selection, 52
  crossovers, 54
  crossovers, MAGIC study, 54
  dichotomous, yes-or-no outcome, 49, 51
  dilution, 46, 47, 53
  dilution (including crossovers), 53–55
  effect measurement, 49–51
  effect size, 46, 53
  efficacy, interim looks, 46

Index **197**

endpoint types, 46
equivalence, noninferiority trials, 60–61
   on-treatment analysis, 61
   per-protocol analysis, 61
   RECORD trial, 61
experimental group, 55
experimental therapy, 52
figuring effect size, 51–52
follow-up time, 47
general factors, 47
interim efficacy monitoring, 47
multiple endpoints, 50–51
null hypothesis, 47
power, 46
power (1–β), 47
primary outcome (primary endpoint), 49
primary trial endpoint, 46
sample size, other complex trials, 61–66
   advantages, disadvantages, 65–66
   CATCH trial, 62, 63
   cluster randomized trial, 62
   cluster unit trials, 62–63
   cluster unit trials, REACT trial, 62
   cohort *vs.* cross-sectional design, 62
   crossover trials, 64–66
   DASH trial, 65–66
   dilution effect, 63
   key issues, 62–63
   number of clusters, 62
   outcome level measurement, 62
   repeated measures designs, 64
SHOCK trial, 51–52
significance and power, 46–49
significance level, 45
significance level (α), 45, 47–48, 48*f*, 96
significance level α and power 1–β, 48, 48*f*
software, 66–67
   essential features, 67
   GLMPOWER procedure, 66
   nQuery Advisor, 66
   PASS, 66
   POWER procedure, 66
   R, 66
   SAS, 66
   S-Plus, 66
standard group, 55
subject accrual, 46, 52–53
superiority trial sample size, 55–60
   A-HeFT trial, 56–57
   difference in means, 55–56, 56*f*
   difference in proportions, 57
   hazard ratio, 57–59, 58*f*, 59*f*
   PEACE trial, 59–60
   percentage reduction of *r*, 58
   proportional hazards, 57
   standardized difference (signal-to-noise ratio), 56
time to event, 47, 49, 51
treatment group strategies, 46, 52
trial duration, 46, 53
two means, standard deviation, 47
two proportions, 47
Type I error probability (significance level or α), 47
Type II error probability (β), 47
values, two proportions, 47
SAS. *See* Statistical Analysis System

Schron, Eleanor, 101–115
SDV. *See* Source document verification
Selection bias (subversion), 37–50
Siami, Sandi, 141–149
Signal-to-noise ratio, 56
Significance level (α), 45, 47–48, 48*f*, 96
Site monitoring, 145–147
Site selection, 132–133
Sleeper, Lynn, 71–99
Social Security Administration database, 161
Software, 66–67
SOPs. *See* Standard operating procedures
Source document verification (SDV), 145
Specimen volumes, 88
Standard deviation, 47
Standard error, 93
Standard operating procedures (SOPs), 143
Standardized difference. *See* Signal-to-noise ratio
Statistical Analysis System (SAS), 66
Study organization and governance, 117–140
   communication, promotion, 137–138
   conclusion, 138
   CTAs, 121–122
   ethics committees, 122–124
   EU, 119
   ICH GCP, 120
   IDE, 121
   IMP, 121
   IND, 121
   investigator, educator meetings, 137
   IRBs, 123
   launch meetings, 137
   meetings, 137
   MHRA, 122
   multisite trial organization, 120–124
   national websites, 122
   protocol finalization, 132
   regulatory agencies, clinical trial authorizations, 120–122
   review boards, 122–124
   site evaluation, 133–134
   site selection, 132–133
   subject recruitment plans, 134–136
      physician attitudes, 136
      site enthusiasm, 136
      subject apprehension, 135
      subject enrollment barriers, 135
   trial design, 136
   trial coordinating center function, organization, 129, 130*f*, 132
      DART trial, 131
      Initio trial, 131
      INSIGHT, 130
      OCC, 130
   trial governance, 124–128, 125*t*
      DMC, 124
      DMC charter, 128
      DMC composition, 127
      DMC composition, DAMOCLES group, 127
      DMC responsibilities, 127
      DMC trials, 126
      Executive Committee, 124
      independent data, safety monitoring committee, 126–127

OCC, 130
PT, 124, 128–129
regulatory imperative, 128
TMG, 124, 128–129
trial stoppage decision, 127
TSC, 124
Tuskegee Syphilis Study, 122
Subgroup analyses, 86–88
Subject attrition, 88
Subject exclusion, 90
Subject follow-up rules, missing data, 152, 154–155, 157–160
Subversion (selection bias), 37–50
Surrogate endpoints, 167–174
  background, 168
  biological, 168
  clinical, 168
  clinical endpoint statistical relationship, 168–169
  conclusion, 172
  definition, 168
  failure reasons, 171, 171*t*
  implementation, 172
  mechanical, 168
  Prentice criteria, 169
  scope, 168–172, 171*t*
  standardized classification system, 168

Tian, Xin, 45–70
TMG. *See* Trial Management Group
Torgerson, David, 27–44
Treatment crossovers, 80
Treatment dilution, 90
Treatment efficacy, 73, 77
Treatment group, 46, 52, 80
Trial endpoints, 79
Trial governance, 124–128
Trial Management Group (TMG), 124
Trial Steering Committee (TSC), 124
TSC. *See* Trial Steering Committee
Tuskegee Syphilis Study, 122

Unit of analysis, 6, 17
Unit of treatment, 17

VAlHeFT. *See* Valsartan Heart Failure Trial
Validity, 10, 20–21, 84
Valsartan Heart Failure Trial (VAlHeFT), 50
Variance, 73, 76, 92

Worst case imputation, 89

NOTES

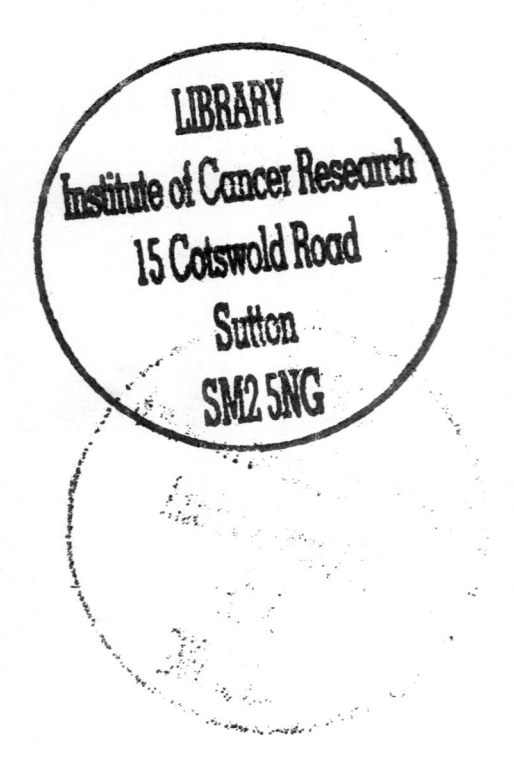

LIBRARY
Institute of Cancer Research
15 Cotswold Road
Sutton
SM2 5NG